BUILD BONE HEALTH

PREVENT AND TREAT OSTEOPOROSIS

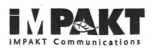

IMPAKT Communications

Health Information Specialists

BUILD BONE HEALTH

PREVENT AND TREAT OSTEOPOROSIS

by

Freedolph Anderson, M.D.

Foreword by Linda Evans

Library of Congress Catalog Card Number: 99-61964
ISBN 1-890694-22-3

Cover design by Tami R. Budz
Linda Evans photograph by Gary Bernstein © 1999

Published by:
IMPAKT Communications, Inc.
P.O. Box 12496
Green Bay, WI 54307-2496
E-mail: impakt@dct.com
Fax: (920) 434-8884
www.impakt.com

Dedication

This book is dedicated to the millions of women and men who are boldly taking charge of their own health and vitality.

Acknowledgments

Many individuals committed to women's health education were involved in the creation of this book. First, a special thank you to actress Linda Evans for writing the foreword and helping to promote osteoporosis awareness. Linda has been using her star-status to educate women about their healthcare choices.

I would also like to extend my gratitude to the people of IMPAKT Communications, Inc., who worked on this project. A special thanks to Karolyn A. Gazella, president of the company, who helped gather research on the topic and coordinate this project. Thanks also to the IMPAKT editor, Frances E. FitzGerald.

Pharmacist Steven Lee has been instrumental in bringing ipriflavone to the United States marketplace. His scientific input on this project was appreciated. Mr. Lee is from Technical Sourcing International, makers of Ostivone™ brand ipriflavone, a dietary supplement ingredient. Thanks also to Susan Brown, Ph.D., Ronald Hoffman, M.D., and the many other scientists and physicians who provided information for this book. And finally, my gratitude to those researchers who have devoted their careers to discovering better osteoporosis treatment and prevention options.

—Freedolph Anderson, M.D.

Foreword

BY LINDA EVANS

While I was involved with the television program *Dynasty*, Congress asked me to speak on the topic of physical fitness. They wanted to motivate individuals to participate in a healthier lifestyle, with the hopes of eventually reducing the financial burden on our unhealthy healthcare system. "What's your secret?" they asked me. "How do you discipline yourself to work out every day?" At the time, my answer was quite simply "survival." In my industry, if you're not physically fit, someone who looks healthier is just around the corner to take your place.

After *Dynasty*, I rebelled against the Hollywood pressures of looking good. I stopped working out and gained about 25 pounds. It was then that I realized that my motivation to work out was all wrong. Today, I exercise and eat right not because I want to look beautiful or need to compete with others, but because I want to *feel* better. After all, we have only one body our entire life. We need to learn how to take care of it.

I speak to women's groups all over the country about the joys of aging. I tell them how they can achieve optimum health, and I confide in them about my own previous lack of knowledge.

When I was in my late 20s, I developed idiopathic edema, which is unexplained water retention. I was given water pills for this condition, which resulted in a calcium/magnesium deficiency that depleted my body of potassium. I was having serious muscle cramps in my feet, legs, and hands. I spent years trying to overcome the problems associated with this deficiency. I took a potassium supplement to help ease the cramping.

Then, I discovered a calcium/magnesium bone-building formula that contained a natural compound called ipriflavone (pronounced i-pri-flay-vone). After taking the product for a few weeks, I noticed that I felt better and the cramps stopped. The ipriflavone actually helps my body absorb the calcium it needs. I'm still fascinated that a natural substance, available economically, over-the-counter, can actually help rebuild and protect my bones. Today, I no longer need to take extra potassium.

Osteoporosis is a key emphasis of my women's health presentations. Osteoporosis is often referred to as the "silent disease," because even though you don't realize it, it's developing long before you actually show any signs. Many individuals don't know anything is wrong until they end up in the doctor's office with a fracture. People, especially women, need to understand that this is a serious problem that begins early in life. When we're young, we never think we'll have a problem because we have youth on our side. However, a woman begins to lose bone mass after age 30 and during pregnancy and breast-feeding.

Fortunately, you can take simple steps early on to prevent osteoporosis. There is also hope for those of you who have been diagnosed with low bone mass or osteoporosis. These same, easy steps will also benefit you.

In this comprehensive, easy-to-read book, Dr. Freedolph Anderson explains how your diet can rob you of important bone density. It's critical that you learn about nutrition and share that knowledge with your family. Many experts have admitted that food doesn't give us everything we require. They just don't grow it like they used to! We need to find what we're missing and replace it. You wouldn't run your car without replacing the oil periodically. The same is true for diet and nutritional supplements. Added nutrients help ensure your body's "engine" runs smoothly for a lifetime.

Dr. Anderson also discusses why exercise is vital to bone health, and describes other lifestyle factors that can either build or damage bones. In addition, you'll learn about the exciting scientific discovery, ipriflavone, and how it can benefit bone health.

Who should read this book? If you have a family history of osteoporosis, have one or more of the risk factors, or want to ensure that you have strong bones for a lifetime, this book will be incredibly valuable. I suggest giving your daughter or granddaughter a copy as well.

I received my wake-up call when I gained weight and discovered I really knew very little about the care and health of my own body. I certainly wasn't ready to give up feeling vital and active.

At age 56, I'm living my life with zest and vitality. Will you be like me—dancing, laughing, running, and shopping until you're 92 years old? Or, will you be bed-ridden or in a chair, watching life pass you by? It's important to take responsibility for things you have control over, or you could find yourself a victim of your own lack of knowledge. Books like this one will help you on your journey toward great health and vitality for a lifetime. Congratulations, Dr. Anderson and IMPAKT Communications.

In good health, always!
Linda Evans
actress and women's health advocate

Contents

"...one in two women will be affected by osteoporosis..."

Introduction

THE SILENT EPIDEMIC

The dictionary defines the term "epidemic" as affecting or tending to affect a disproportionately large number of individuals within a population, community, or region at the same time; spreading rapidly; excessively prevalent. The term is most commonly used in the health field to describe a virus or other infectious condition that is multiplying at a rapid rate. Of course, such occurrences cause understandable concern.

In the early 1990s, the AIDS epidemic rose to a fever pitch as the number of AIDS deaths doubled in a very short period of time. Nearly a decade later, we are faced with another insidious epidemic. It's the silent epidemic of osteoporosis. Its damaging health impact cannot be denied.

A key component to any health epidemic is its "rapid spread and excessive prevalence." Certainly, these alarming statistics paint a sobering picture of osteoporosis:

✔ According to the National Institutes of Health, in 1984, osteoporosis cost the United States less than $4 billion annually. Just 11 years later, the National Osteoporosis Foundation estimated that direct expenditures due to osteoporosis and associated fractures cost the United States nearly $14 billion. That's $38 million a day!

✔ Today, 10 million Americans have osteoporosis and another 18 million have low bone mass, which places them at high risk of developing osteoporosis.

✔ After the age of 50, one-half of all women and one in eight men will eventually develop an osteoporosis-related fracture.

✔ More than 1.5 million fractures occur each year as a result of osteoporosis.

✔ Of the 300,000 people experiencing hip fractures annually, 50 percent will never walk without assistance again, and up to 30 percent will be unable to live independently. Another 25 percent will die within one year.

✔ A woman's risk of developing a hip fracture is equal to the risk of developing breast, ovarian, and uterine cancer *combined.*

✔ The National Osteoporosis Foundation has predicted that if left unchecked, by the year 2015, 41 million people will be diagnosed with osteoporosis or low bone mass. That's nearly a 50 percent increase in only 15 years.

Yes, we have an epidemic on our hands. It's amazing that although osteoporosis will affect one in two women, we hear very little about the dangers of this condition. However, as we enter the new millennium, we can no longer stay silent about this disease. If we are to reverse this damaging trend, we must become familiar with the enemy. Protecting our bone health should be a key concern for all of us who want to live life with vitality.

Bone structure should be a primary concern of any viable health program. A strong frame provides an important foundation to build on. Fortunately, there are many ways you can protect your inner foundation, using techniques that are well within your reach.

Interested in prevention?

This book was written for two groups of people:

1. Those interested in preventing osteoporosis and maintaining strong bone health for a lifetime.
2. Those who have been diagnosed with osteoporosis or low bone mass.

First, a message to readers interested in keeping their bones strong and preventing osteoporosis.

You will gain much benefit from the bone-building program outlined in this book. The younger you begin the program, the better your chance of maintaining peak bone health for your entire life. Your proactive approach will help ensure that your bone structure supports you and your active lifestyle as you age.

While there are no guarantees in health or in life, you can improve your own bone health. The odds are in your favor if you participate in an active bone-building program while you still have strong bones. Congratulations for taking this important first step. The results you achieve will confirm that your time and energy were well spent.

Do you have osteoporosis or low bone mass?

It's never too late to incorporate positive bone-building habits into your everyday life. If you've gotten an osteoporosis diagnosis, or low bone mass test result, it is more important than ever that you pay close attention to the advice presented here.

But remember, this information is for educational purposes only. I do not encourage self-diagnosis or self-treatment. If you are presently taking a prescription medication, do not discontinue your treatment without first consulting your doctor.

Osteoporosis is a serious condition that requires the care of a trained physician. Look for a physician who is willing to work with you to create a comprehensive treatment plan. I encourage you to give this book to your doctor for his/her review. Scientific references are provided at the back of the book.

My intention is to provide a comprehensive overview of osteoporosis; however, keep in mind that circumstances can vary dramatically from one individual to the next. If you have questions after reading any part of this book, please discuss your concerns with your physician. Informa-tion is power, and knowledge is your best ally in your fight to preserve or regain your health. Never be afraid to ask questions and search for answers that are specific to your individual situation.

Ending the silence

As a specialist in obstetrics and gynecology, I have researched the topic of bone health extensively. The information for this book has been taken from my own educational and clinical experiences, as well as from a variety of professional sources. The goal of this book is to provide you with a clear view of all of your options and to help end the silence surrounding osteoporosis and bone health. Together, we can help put an end to this silent epidemic.

For your convenience, I have provided you with some terms on the next page. You may want to familiarize yourself with these descriptions before you read on.

Terms you should know:

Bone mineral density (BMD) = Calcium content of the bone.

Bone mass = Total amount of bone tissue.

Calcitonin = Hormone secreted by the thyroid gland that inhibits bone breakdown.

Estrogen = A group of hormones produced primarily in the ovaries.

Genetic peak bone mass = Total maximum amount of bone achieved prior to age 30 when bone mass begins to decline.

Ipriflavone = An isoflavone, which is a compound that naturally occurs in plants and foods.

Isoflavone = A natural compound found in plants that has estogenic properties.

Menopause = When the ovaries stop making eggs and menstruation stops.

Osteoblast = Cells that help re-build bone tissue.

Osteoclast = Cells that help break down bone and clear out old or deformed bone tissue.

Osteopenia = Decreased BMD, not yet affecting fracture rate.

Osteoporosis = Decreased BMD and changes in bone structure, making bones frail and easily fractured.

Parathyroid = Small endocrine gland, located close to the thyroid, that produces a hormone involved in calcium utilization.

"...because bone is living tissue, it is affected by outside influences..."

Chapter One

BONE STRUCTURE

A builder or architect would certainly understand the importance of the human skeleton. Our skeletal system creates the framework for our bodies, just as the frame of a building holds the brick and mortar in place. Without a solid frame, the infrastructure of our entire lives would crumble.

Consider the flurry of physical movements that encompasses our daily lives. How many times have you stood up today? Or bent over to pick up something? Reached for the telephone?

From baking to basketball, hugs to handshakes, vacuuming to vacationing, physical movement requires healthy bone structure. You even relied on your bone structure to pick up and read this book. And yet, so many of us take our bones for granted. After all, bones are simply hard, lifeless support beams that we hang the important stuff on, right? Wrong!

In fact, as you read this page, your bones are undergoing an important, ever-changing remodeling process. Bone is living tissue that constantly regenerates itself. Bone mass refers to the amount and thickness of the bone. The more bone mass you have, the stronger your bones are.

Two types of bone cells are responsible for reshaping and changing bone structure and creating healthy bone mass. Osteoclast cells circulate and detect older and/or damaged bone materials. Osteoclasts then dissolve the unwanted material, leaving a space in the bone. This process is known as the bone resorption phase (refer to the illustration on page 8).

During the reversal phase, osteoblast cells move into the vacant space. Osteoblast cells then produce new bone tissue to

Bone Remodeling

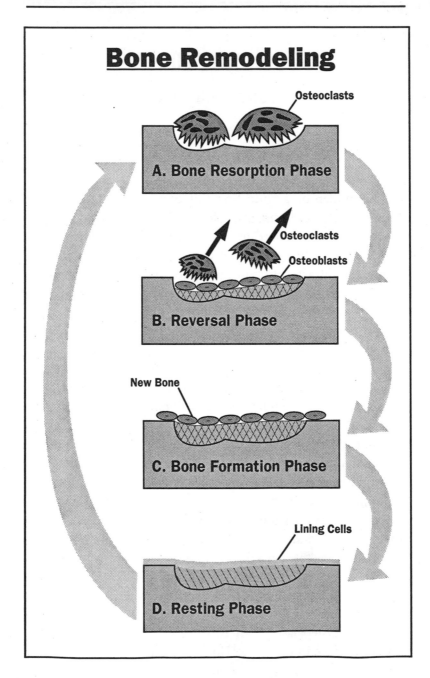

Osteoclasts

A. Bone Resorption Phase

Osteoclasts

Osteoblasts

B. Reversal Phase

New Bone

C. Bone Formation Phase

Lining Cells

D. Resting Phase

fill in the gap, which is known as the bone formation-phase. Prior to osteoclast activity, there is a resting phase. And this cycle is repeated countless times during our lifetime. Think of it this way: Osteoblasts (with a "b") *build* bone tissue, while osteoclasts (with a "c") *clear* out old bone tissue.

In healthy, premenopausal women, the rate of bone resorption and bone formation are very similar. Therefore, if bone resorption speeds up for some reason, then healthy bone makes up for it by increasing the amount of new bone.

This sophisticated, internal control mechanism ensures that bone health remains fairly constant. It's an "out with the old, in with the new" mentality that keeps bones healthy and strong. In fact, every eight years, we have an entirely new skeleton!

Unfortunately, as we age, this process becomes unbalanced. Bone tissue begins to break down faster than new bone tissue can be made. Osteoblast activity can't keep up with osteoclast activity.

Bone density tests are available that can evaluate your rate of bone loss. They can help determine your risk of fractures, and detect osteoporosis before you ever fracture a bone. The bone densitometry, using an X-ray technique, is presently the most common type of test.

"Although the test itself has limitations, it can be very reassuring for many women," explains renowned women's wellness doctor Christiane Northrup, M.D., and author of *Women's Bodies, Women's Wisdom*. "I recommend this for those women who need more data before deciding on hormone therapy, who need motivation to change their diets and start exercising, and who have a family history of osteoporosis."

By the age of 20, the average female has about 98 percent of her bone mass. Peak bone mass is achieved at age 30. After age 30, bone is lost at an average rate of 0.4 percent per year. With menopause, women lose about two percent of the outer layer of bone and five percent of the inner spongy tissue of the bone per year for the first five to eight years. After that, it stabilizes at 0.4 percent again.

Fortunately, because bone is living tissue, outside influences—such as diet and other lifestyle factors—can affect it. This means that, given the right environment, bones can actually heal themselves or regenerate.

The National Osteoporosis Foundation provides this vivid analogy: "Think of your bones as a savings account. There is only as much bone mass in your account as you deposit."

Later we will learn how we can directly influence our individual bone "savings account."

Bone structure basics

Unfortunately, the closest most people have come to bone health education is the chanting of the folk song: "The hip bone's connected to the leg bone…" It would be nice if it were that simple. The reality is, bone health is very complex.

While it may not be important to know the difference between the clavicle and scapula—which are both a part of the pectoral section of the skeleton—it is critical that we recognize the importance of our bone structure.

In addition to constantly remodeling to remain strong, our bones serve many other important purposes, including:

✔ Protecting vital internal organs.
✔ Providing structural support for muscles.
✔ Serving as points of attachment for muscles, which create levers, making movement possible.

And then there is the important task of housing bone marrow. Bone marrow is the soft material that fills the bone cavity. Bone marrow produces red blood cells, B-cells and T-cells, important components of our immune system. These cells help the body fight illness and disease. Researchers are discovering an intricate relationship between bone activity and the immune system. It's easy to see why bone health is so important to overall health.

The Human Skeleton

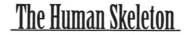

- **206 BONES IN ALL**

- **24 VERTEBRAE**

- **24 RIBS**

- **14 BONES IN THE FACE**

- **3 SMALL BONES IN THE EARS**

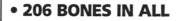

The estrogen connection

Hormones play a vital role in the development of bone. The most well-known hormone for bone health is estrogen. Estrogen actually represents a group of hormones consisting of estriol, estrone, and estradiol. While the issue of estrogen replacement is quite controversial, the physiology of estrogen and bone formation is not. Estrogen prevents rapid bone resorption and can help slow the rate of bone loss. Estrogen does not, however, increase bone formation. There is some evidence that it may, but its main mechanism of action is decreasing resorption.

Estrogen influences osteoclast cell activity. And remember, it's the osteoclasts that clear out damaged or dead bone cells, creating that vacancy for new bone tissue.

The female body manufactures estrogen primarily in the ovaries. Women continue to produce small amounts of estrogen after menopause by converting adrenal and ovarian androgens in the fat to estrogen. Yes, the ovaries continue to produce androgens after menopause.

Many health experts believe that estrogen works very closely with progesterone, another hormone produced in the ovaries. Similar to the way calcium and magnesium work together, estrogen and progesterone seem to form a strong partnership.

The extent to which progesterone can promote bone health is not yet understood. Researchers at the University of Toronto concluded (*J Prosthet Dent*, Jan 1998) that "...progesterone replacement therapy has been shown to prevent postmenopausal bone loss associated with ovarian dysfunction." And yet, Japanese researchers reported in the journal *Bone* that "...progesterone alone cannot prevent bone loss or the increase in turnover after oopherectomy (i.e., surgical removal of one or both ovaries) and that estrogen, not progesterone, accounted for all of the bone activity in this study."

We will find that progesterone is just one small part of the overall bone health picture. Prescription progesterone is often used with estrogen to offset uterine cancer risks in menopausal women.

In men, and to some degree in women, testosterone affects bone health. The male body converts testosterone into estrogen. It is believed that one of the reasons men do not succumb to osteoporosis as readily as women do is that they manufacture hormones their entire lives, while women stop producing estrogen at menopause.

All three of these hormones play a critical role in our overall health. They work both independently and synergistically to help influence many body functions, including bone health. Modern technology allows your physician to determine your exact hormone levels.

In addition to estrogen, progesterone, and testosterone, parathyroid hormones, secreted by glands in the neck, also contribute to bone health. Parathyroid hormones directly control and balance calcium stores in the body. In a later chapter, we will discover the importance of the mineral calcium to bone health.

In his book, *The Osteoporosis Solution*, Carl Germano, R.D., C.N.S., explains that the parathyroid hormone increases blood calcium levels "first, by telling the kidneys to return more calcium to the bloodstream instead of excreting it, and second, by breaking down bone to release calcium."

The result is balanced calcium levels in the body, which is important to overall bone health. "The delicate balance between osteoclasts that break down bone, osteoblasts that build up bone, and hormones that regulate their activity, underscores bone's importance to all the body's systems," explains Germano.

Chapter highlights:

- Bone is living tissue that "turns over" and changes on a daily basis.
- Diet and lifestyle factors either negatively or positively affect bone tissue.
- The two types of bone cells involved in bone regeneration and formation are known as osteoclast and osteoblast cells. Osteoclasts clear out old or damaged cells, while osteoblasts fill in the gaps to help build new bone tissue. This is known as bone remodeling.
- The human skeleton serves many important purposes, such as storing bone marrow, protecting vital organs, supporting muscles, and allowing movement.
- Hormones, such as estrogen, progesterone, testosterone, and parathyroid hormone, all play key roles in bone development.

"Osteoporosis is a disabling and sometimes deadly disease..."

Chapter Two
OSTEOPOROSIS OVERVIEW

Imagine leaning over to grab a gallon of ice cream from the grocery store freezer and breaking a rib. Imagine fracturing your wrist as you shut the car door. A simple fall on the ice, or just twisting differently as you get out of bed, can cause a hip fracture. These are typical ways individuals find out they have osteoporosis. A simple life activity that they've done hundreds, perhaps thousands, of times in their life, suddenly causes them to break a bone. This is osteoporosis and its outcome can be devastating.

According to the National Institutes of Health Consensus Development Conference on Osteoporosis, "A fall, blow, or lifting action that would not bruise or strain the average person can easily cause one or more bones to break in a person with severe osteoporosis."

Osteoporosis is a disabling and sometimes deadly disease, characterized by progressive loss of bone mass and bone strength. Bones become fragile and are much more likely to break. These broken bones—also called fractures—are the most dangerous outcome of osteoporosis. Any bone can fracture; however, the most common sites are the hip, spine, and wrist. The hip and spine are the most serious.

A hip fracture almost always requires hospitalization and major surgery, explains the National Osteoporosis Foundation. This injury can impair a person's ability to walk without aid, and may cause prolonged or permanent disability. Spinal or vertebral fractures also have serious consequences, including loss of height, severe back pain, and deformity.

As you may recall, 25 percent of individuals who experience

Fractures:
THE MOST DANGEROUS OUTCOME OF OSTEOPOROSIS

There are three major types of fractures that can occur in an individual with osteoporosis:

Vertebral: This is when one or more vertebrae in the spine becomes weak and collapses. This can occur simply as a result of the body's own weight, or perhaps after lifting even a small object. Because most of these fractures happen on the front side of the vertebrae, the spine caves downward, resulting in a hunched-over posture.

Hip: This is the most serious type of fracture and can result in permanent disability or even death. Due to osteoporosis, and the fact that the hip bone is more rigid to begin with, it often takes only a small trauma to the area to result in a fracture.

Wrist: Often the result of a fall, this fracture occurs just above the wrist as the hand is placed backward and outward. It is just as common as hip fractures; however, it is not nearly as serious.

a hip fracture die within one year of the break. This is due to medical complications and a general failure to thrive.

The stooped posture, and more than one to two inches of lost height, indicate that osteoporosis has attacked the spine. This is due to vertebral fractures. A "dowager's hump" may develop, a manifestation of the slow, painless loss of bone mass in the neck/upper spine area.

In an October 1997 update on primary osteoporosis, Mayo Clinic researchers concluded: "Osteoporosis is the most common bone disorder encountered in clinical practice. It is also one of the most important diseases facing our aging population."

A quick history lesson

While fragile bones have been discussed in the medical literature for hundreds of years, it wasn't until after World War I that osteoporosis began to attract attention. Was this newfound focus due to an increased life span and more sophisticated testing methods, or was osteoporosis on the rise? Much evidence indicates that osteoporosis is more common in today's society than ever before.

"...increasing attention to osteoporosis in the early twentieth century was due, at least in part, to an increased prevalence of the condition," explains Dr. Gaby in his book, *Preventing and Reversing Osteoporosis*. "The possibility that osteoporosis is largely a disease of modern civilization is supported by recent epidemiologic studies from Europe."

According to a 1993 article featured in the European medical journal, *The Lancet*, scientists compared skeletal bone mass from two centuries ago with modern-day women. They found bone loss was much more significant in contemporary women than their centuries-old counterparts, providing even more proof that osteoporosis is—at least in part—a disease of our modern times.

According to a recently published article in a European rheumatology medical journal (*Baillieres Clin Rheumatol* Aug

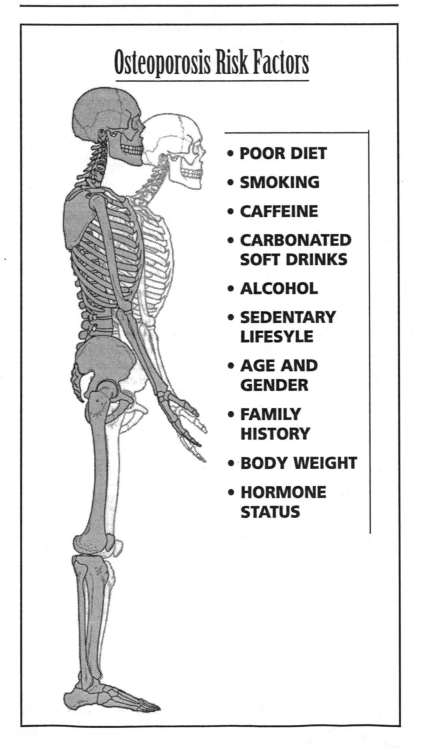

Osteoporosis Risk Factors

- **POOR DIET**
- **SMOKING**
- **CAFFEINE**
- **CARBONATED SOFT DRINKS**
- **ALCOHOL**
- **SEDENTARY LIFESYLE**
- **AGE AND GENDER**
- **FAMILY HISTORY**
- **BODY WEIGHT**
- **HORMONE STATUS**

1997), just 10 years ago, the word osteoporosis did not exist in the vocabulary of the general public throughout Europe. The authors revealed that "The majority of doctors had dismissed osteoporosis as a normal process of aging, affecting only the very elderly, and about which nothing could be done." Today, Europeans have embarked upon a substantial awareness program designed to clarify this misconception.

Researchers from the University of Colorado Health Sciences Center in Denver concluded in the Summer 1998 edition of the journal *Menopause* that "...osteoporosis should no longer be an accepted process of aging."

Today, organizations in the United States, such as the National Osteoporosis Foundation and the Osteoporosis Education Project, are working diligently to educate the general public about osteoporosis. (For more information about these organizations, refer to Appendix I on page 78.)

Causes and risk factors

If osteoporosis is a disease associated with our modern-day living, then its causes, in part, can be traced to modern-day lifestyle factors. It has been hypothesized that nutritional and dietary changes, coupled with environmental factors (e.g., increased toxins in the air, food, and water), are contributing to the increase in osteoporosis. Dr. Gaby theorizes that chronic, low-level deficiencies of a wide range of micronutrients may increase the risk of developing this condition.

From a physiological standpoint, we know that a decrease in estrogen production, typically associated with menopause, can lead to osteoporosis. While estrogen deficiency is a contributor, we also know that bone loss begins long before menopause.

"...up to 50 percent of the bone that women lose over their life span is lost before menopause even begins," according to Dr. Northrup. "Statistics show that six percent to 18 percent of women between 25 and 35 years of age have abnormally low bone density."

Dr. Northrup concludes that loss of bone mass is more complicated than simply a loss of estrogen. In fact, I am sure we will eventually discover a complex synergism between diet, lifestyle factors, hormones, and isolated nutrients that provide the most appropriate osteoporosis prevention plan. Chapter three will cover the major impact of diet on overall bone health.

Here is a brief description of some other direct causes of osteoporosis:

- ✔ Hyperparathyroidism, which is excess secretion of the parathyroid hormone.
- ✔ An overactive thyroid gland.
- ✔ Cushing's syndrome, which is excess secretion of adrenal hormones.
- ✔ Prescription drug use, particularly cortisone and prednisone, aluminum-containing antacids, anticonvulsants, and thyroid medications. Talk to your doctor if you're wondering whether your prescription medication will interfere with the health of your bones.

Besides a poor diet, the following lifestyle habits will accelerate bone loss and promote osteoporosis: (Positive lifestyle and dietary habits will be covered in chapter three.)

- ✔ **Smoking.** The dangerous health effects of smoking have long been established. The connection between smoking and bone loss has not been so clear. It is known, however, that nicotine causes poor calcium absorption and has an anti-estrogen effect.
- ✔ **Caffeine.** Coffee, cola soft drinks, chocolate, and other caffeine-containing beverages and foods sap calcium from the body. This mineral is vital to proper bone formation. Interestingly, in one study featured in a 1994 issue of the *American Journal of Clinical Nutrition*,

caffeine-consuming women whose calcium intake was high did not have as much bone loss as the women who had low calcium intakes. The researchers concluded that two to three cups of brewed coffee each day accelerates bone loss in women who are not getting enough calcium.

✔ **Alcohol.** Excessive alcohol intake poses many dangerous health problems, among them the development of osteoporosis. Clinical studies on moderate to low alcohol intake and bone health have not yet been done.

✔ **Sedentary lifestyle.** Numerous studies have shown that regular exercise builds bone mass, and that a sedentary lifestyle can contribute to osteoporosis. However, keep in mind that the opposite extreme is also potentially harmful. Excessive exercise can reduce body fat (where some estrogen is made and stored) and negatively affect hormone balance. Clearly, however, the benefits of moderate, consistent physical activity far outweigh any drawbacks.

The Study of Osteoporotic Fractures (SOF), funded by the National Institute of Arthritis and Musculoskeletal and Skin Diseases and the National Institute on Aging, assessed a variety of risk factors, including bone mass, in more than 9,500 women, age 65 and older, who had not had a previous hip fracture. They found that the impact of the individual risk factors is not nearly as great as the combination of risk factors. Specifically regarding hip fracture, the study found that "...maintaining body weight, walking for exercise, avoiding long-acting benzodiazepines (for anxiety and insomnia), minimizing caffeine intake, and treating impaired visual function are among the steps that may decrease the risk of hip fracture."

As with other conditions, certain individuals face a higher risk of osteoporosis than others. Following are the key osteoporosis risk factors:

✔ **Age and gender.** The older you are, the more likely you are to develop osteoporosis. In addition, women develop this condition four times more than men do.

✔ **Genetics.** A family history of osteoporosis, especially a parent, increases your chances of developing this condition. Population studies have shown that up to 85 percent of the variance in bone mass is genetically determined. Remember, however, that a family history or genetic predisposition doesn't mean this condition is inevitable for you. You will still benefit greatly from the program outlined in this book.

✔ **Bone structure and body weight.** This is one of those cases where it's better to carry a little extra weight. Studies have shown that thin women with small bone structure are at a higher risk of developing osteoporosis.

✔ **Hormone status.** Normal or early menopause increases the risk of osteoporosis. Menstrual cycle irregularities and other hormonal imbalances can also lead to osteoporosis. It is widely known that female athletes (specifically gymnasts and ballet dancers, who are typically thin and small-boned) are more likely to develop low bone mass. In addition, eating disorders, such as anorexia and bulimia, can cause hormonal imbalances that lead to osteoporosis.

✔ **Race.** According to a recent report by the National Osteoporosis Risk Assessment study, Asian, Native American, and Latino women face a higher risk of developing this condition than Caucasian women do. African American women appear to have the lowest risk of osteoporosis.

✔ **Medications and certain illnesses.** Cortisone and other drugs can cause osteoporosis. It can also develop as a result of illnesses causing immobilization, endocrine disorders such as overactive thyroid, and rheumatoid arthritis. Young adult survivors of childhood cancers are predisposed to osteopenia (i.e., decreased bone mineral density).

✔ **Lifestyle.** The following factors increase your risk of developing osteoporosis:
—Smoking
—Alcohol and caffeine intake
—Lack of physical activity
—Poor diet, with little emphasis on calcium-containing foods

As you can see, many of these factors are well within your control. Reducing your risk means choosing healthier lifestyle activities.

Conventional treatment

Many patients with osteoporosis don't even realize they have the condition until they experience their first bone fracture. At that time, a bone density test provides an accurate diagnosis and determines the extent of the problem (refer to page 26). A typical X-ray does not provide a definitive diagnosis of osteoporosis. Proper diagnosis is critical.

A fairly new testing technique measures bone resorption (i.e., bone breakdown) via a urine sample. This test—known as the NTx Osteomark—is gaining popularity among clinicians. The Osteoporosis Education Project, directed by Susan Brown, Ph.D., uses the NTx Osteomark in its research and is presently exploring the full value of this test in clinical practice. "This urine marker of bone breakdown has the potential to uniquely distinguish if bone loss is currently on-going or if bone is currently stable," explains Dr. Brown.

If the accuracy of the test is confirmed, it will definitely provide a more convenient, less expensive way to evaluate risk and determine if a particular therapy is working.

Diagnostic Methods
BONE DENSITY TESTS

Physicians use different tests to determine bone mass and help predict risk of fracture. Each test has advantages and disadvantages. Your physician will choose the test(s) most appropriate for your individual situation. They include:

Dual-energy X-ray absorptiometry (DXA, DEXA)

Quantitative computed tomography

Radiographic absorptiometry (RA)

Single-energy X-ray absorptiometry (SXA)

Ultrasound densitometry

As with most illnesses, early diagnosis contributes greatly to the success of any treatment plan. Individuals who are at high risk should ask their doctor about a bone density test. If caught early, osteoporosis is treatable. Certainly, you will discover that it is also largely preventable. It is important to be aware of your body. Without becoming paranoid, pay close attention to how you feel physically as you move through your day. See your doctor if you are at high risk of developing osteoporosis (refer to risk assessment Appendix II on page 80).

According to the journal, *Spine*, researchers explain, "In the development of osteoporosis, there is often a long latent period before the appearance of the main clinical manifestation, pathologic fractures. The earliest symptom of osteoporosis is often an episode of acute back pain caused by a pathologic vertebral compression fracture, or an episode of groin or thigh pain caused by a pathologic hip fracture."

That's why osteoporosis is referred to as the "silent disease," because it develops quietly over the years until it arrives, literally crashing in on its victim. This is really a condition that has its roots in childhood.

Conventional medical practitioners treat osteoporosis primarily with prescription medications, while encouraging the use of a calcium supplement or a higher calcium diet. We will address the calcium and diet issue in the next chapter. Now, let's take a closer look at the four medications presently approved in the United States for the prevention and/or treatment of osteoporosis.

❶ **Estrogen.** Estrogen replacement therapy, using prescription estrogen, is probably the most common conventional medicine used to prevent and treat osteoporosis. From a purely physiological standpoint, estrogen is really an effective treatment for osteoporosis. However, its use remains controversial. Susan E. Brown, Ph.D., author of *Better Bones, Better Bodies*, is one of many professionals who feels osteoporosis is a complicated condition that we've tried to turn into a simple problem of estrogen deficiency. No matter which side of the "estrogen fence" you're on, the fact remains that it is a medication that can cause problems for some women.

Side effects of estrogen replacement therapy include withdrawal bleeding, fluid retention, bloating, headache, nausea, anxiety, irritability, vaginal discharge, and others. In addition, many women are concerned about their increased risk of developing breast cancer (the increased uterine cancer risk can be alleviated with simultaneous progesterone therapy). For these reasons, many women who begin estrogen therapy stop taking their medication within only a few months of use. According to a 1991 issue of the *British Journal of General Practice*, only five percent of women receiving estrogen said they requested it. In that same issue, 80 percent of those women on estrogen reportedly said they would have liked more information. Clearly, the estrogen controversy is far from over.

❷ **Bisphosphonates (trade name Fosamax™).** In clinical trials, this medication did help slow bone loss and reduced fracture risk. Unfortunately, many people have difficulty taking the medication because it causes serious gastrointestinal problems, especially involving the esophagus. Because of this problem, the patient must take the medication first thing in the morning on an empty stomach, cannot lie down for at least 30 minutes after taking it, and can't have anything to eat or drink during that time.

According to the *Physician's Desk Reference*, the esophageal irritations can become so severe that ulcers may form, sometimes requiring hospitalization. A recent study published in the *Journal of Managed Care Pharmacy* (October 1998) found that gastrointestinal problems associated with Fosamax usage occurred far more frequently than reported in clinical trials. "Nearly one in three women using alendronate (i.e., Fosamax) daily to treat osteoporosis complained of new upper gastrointestinal symptoms...Of that group, 46 percent discontinued use of the drug within 10 months..." Senior investigator of the study, Bruce Ettinger, M.D., concluded that physicians "should really think twice" before giving their patients Fosamax.

According to a 1998 press release on Fosamax, it is the top-selling drug *solely* used for osteoporosis in the United States, controlling about one-half of the market. Usually, women who will not or cannot take estrogen resort to taking Fosamax. Unfortunately, they often find this is not a feasible alternative.

❸ **Selective Estrogen Receptor Modulators (SERMS).** This is a new class of osteoporosis drugs. The most popular one is raloxifene, trade name Evista™. These drugs act like estrogen on some levels, but supposedly do not stimulate uterine or breast tissue, which can lead to cancer. However, one of the problems with raloxifene is that it blocks estrogen receptors in the brain, and that's where hot flashes are controlled. As a result, many women on raloxifene experience severe hot flashes. As with estrogen, blood clots can also occur with this drug. Effects on ovarian activity in younger women are not known at this time.

❹ **Calcitonin.** Calcitonin is a hormone produced in the thyroid and thymus glands. It stimulates the movement of calcium from the blood to the bones. Remember, if the bones don't get enough calcium, they weaken. While studies have shown that calcitonin can slow bone loss, its effects on fracture reduction have not been proven. Key side effects of calcitonin include nosebleeds, allergic reactions, and nausea. Previously, calcitonin was only available by injection, which made it quite inconvenient and costly. Today, calcitonin is available in a nasal spray. It cannot be taken orally because it is a protein, and is digested before it can begin to work.

Researchers from Belgium recently concluded (*Endocrinol Metab Clin North Am*, June 1998) that "None of the currently available medications for osteoporosis have demonstrated the ability to fully prevent the occurrence of new vertebral or peripheral osteoporotic fractures once the disease is established."

Based on my own clinical experiences and information from other physicians, various side effects make it difficult for many women to comply with these therapies. Obviously, if an individual cannot tolerate the medication, he/she will stop taking it. At that point, the medication is useless. In addition to the side effects, the long-term effects of some of these drugs are not fully understood.

Dr. Brown believes these drugs have "detrimental drawbacks that make them less than ideal, and none of them are terribly effective." It is important to point out, however, that all of these drugs have been clinically evaluated and are accepted as osteoporosis treatments by the Food and Drug Administration (FDA), who approves new drugs in the United States.

Several other drugs are currently being investigated for the treatment and prevention of osteoporosis. Presently, studies are underway on a new class of drugs for osteoporosis, utilizing recombinant (i.e., gene-splicing technique) parathyroid hormone.

With increased awareness of this condition comes increased pressure to find a medical solution. As we will discover in the next chapter, there is not likely to be a single "magic bullet." A condition this complex and widespread requires a more comprehensive approach to ensure consistent results.

If we are to successfully fight this growing epidemic, we must focus our efforts on safe, effective ways to maximize genetic peak bone mass and minimize bone loss. The treatment plan that can do that, without risky side effects, will be the plan that is most accepted by the medical community and embraced by the general public.

In the next chapter, we will discover that Mother Nature has provided us with some of the most effective solutions to the osteoporosis dilemma.

Test Your Knowledge...

TRUE OR FALSE?

Circle the appropriate response. Answers appear in the chapter highlights section on the next page.

1. Osteoporosis begins developing after age 50.
   True   False

2. Men can also get osteoporosis.
   True   False

3. The first sign of this disease is often a bone fracture.
   True   False

4. It is uncommon for osteoporosis to cause a fracture of the spine.
   True   False

5. You can still prevent this disease, even if your mother has osteoporosis.
   True   False

6. The three most common sites for a fracture are the spine, hip, and wrist.
   True   False

7. Drinking alcohol does not increase the risk of developing osteoporosis.
   True   False

8. Bones are living tissue that regenerate regularly.
   True   False

Chapter highlights:

- Osteoporosis is a serious condition that can result in permanent disability or even death.
- A key sign of osteoporosis is when bones break during circumstances that would not normally cause a break, such as lifting a fairly light object.
- The three most common, major types of fractures associated with osteoporosis are vertebral, hip, and wrist.
- Many risk factors can increase an individual's chance of developing osteoporosis.
- Menopausal women experience bone loss more rapidly.
- Lifestyle factors within our control can lead to bone loss, including smoking, caffeine intake, and lack of activity, among others.
- Diagnostic measures are available to help track bone density.
- Conventional medicine offers four types of approved drugs to deal with osteoporosis from a prevention or treatment perspective.
- While conventional drugs have been shown to be effective in clinical studies, side effects do occur.

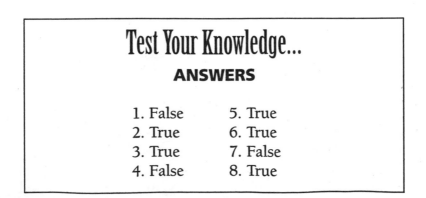

Test Your Knowledge...
ANSWERS

1. False	5. True
2. True	6. True
3. True	7. False
4. False	8. True

"Exercise is perhaps the most powerful medicine available to us today..."

Chapter Three
NATURE'S PLAN

In all of her glory and majesty, Mother Nature has provided many tools we can use to gain good health—including optimum bone health. It was Henry David Thoreau who reminded us: "Nature is doing her best each moment to make us well. She exists for no other end."

Although I am a conventionally trained physician, it has become clear to me that a comprehensive, "natural" approach may provide many benefits in the prevention of osteoporosis. I have evaluated the medical literature and discovered many logical and scientifically sound concepts that are presently labeled "alternative." I have learned to keep an open mind in an effort to analyze what's truly best for the patient and the public at large. While I am disappointed by some of the "alternative" treatment options, unsubstantiated by logic or solid science, I am impressed with some of the concepts and substances with proven benefits.

"Complementary physicians take a broader view with regard to osteoporosis. In addition to confronting the many risk factors long before menopause occurs, they supplement with the full range of nutrients necessary for building bone," states holistic medical doctor and writer Michael Schachter, M.D.

As with all things in life, balance is important. Finding a common ground, a happy medium between two extremes, typically provides the most benefit to patients. This integrative approach will forge new paths in effective patient care in the new millennium. This is especially true for degenerative diseases such as osteoporosis.

It's important to reiterate that the goal of my bone-building program/osteoporosis prevention plan is two-fold:

❶ Maximize genetic peak bone mass.
❷ Minimize bone loss.

Start early!

According to the National Osteoporosis Foundation, "Building strong bones during childhood and adolescence can be the best defense against developing osteoporosis later."

Osteoporosis surfaces in the elderly, but it really is a disease of childhood. Bone health begins early. As you have learned, bone mass reaches its peak when you are about 30 years old. Your diet and lifestyle habits before that age have a dramatic impact on bone health later in life. Young women, especially, should pay attention to their diet. It is critical that teenage girls get enough calcium, magnesium, vitamin D, and other bone-building nutrients in their daily diet.

Researchers at Wayne State University School of Medicine warn, "Parents should be counseled regarding their children's diet and lifestyle to optimize peak adult bone mass and ensure adequate dietary calcium intake. Adults should be counseled to minimize behaviors that result in accelerated bone loss (e.g., smoking, alcohol use, anorexia, bulimia)."

In fact, I encourage you to pass this book on to your daughter, niece, or granddaughter when you're done reading it. Early awareness and prevention is the ultimate bone-building medicine.

With this in mind, let's take a close look at the important components of nature's bone-building plan, including diet, lifestyle factors, and nutritional supplements (i.e., vitamins, minerals, and herbs).

What a difference a diet makes

Thomas Edison predicted that "The doctor of the future will give no medicine, but will interest his patient in the care of the human frame, in diet, and in the cause and prevention of disease." Perhaps Edison was speaking directly about osteoporosis when he referred to the "human frame."

It is difficult to find a doctor who doesn't focus primarily on medications. However, the importance of diet for good health cannot be understated.

Because bone is a living, growing, changing tissue, it can be influenced by diet. In fact, it requires a very specific diet in order to achieve and maintain peak bone mass. In addition, and perhaps the most exciting aspect of osteoporosis, is that it can, in some cases, even be reversed. Best of all, the only "side effect" of using a healthful diet to prevent and treat osteoporosis is better overall health.

Bone tissue has diverse nutritional requirements. It interacts in complex ways with the rest of the body. It is unlikely that the typical American diet could nourish our bones while harming the rest of our body.

Some physicians believe calcium is the only dietary factor that influences bone health. There have not been any broadscale, double-blind studies to determine the exact effect diet has on the development of osteoporosis. However, solid clinical information and anecdotal evidence suggests that diet is more important than previously thought. A balanced diet nourishes the bones with much more than just calcium.

We also know that food processing, additives, and preservatives make our entire food supply less nutritional than in previous decades. For this reason, it is necessary to pay close attention to the quality of the foods we choose.

Before we delve into specific dietary requirements for bone health, let's address "the big three"—carbohydrates, fats, and protein. As we look at each area of the diet, balance is important.

The Typical American Diet

OVERFED AND UNDERNOURISHED?

According to the National Health and Nutritional Examination Survey (NHANES), Americans are not getting enough of at least a dozen essential nutrients. The survey revealed that the typical American consumes the following each year:

- 756 doughnuts
- 60 pounds of cakes and cookies
- 23 gallons of ice cream
- 22 pounds of candy
- 134 pounds of refined sugar
- 482 servings of soft drinks

"Clearly, as a nation, we are ingesting plenty of calories, but precious few nutrients," explains wellness expert Margaret Ames, Ph.D., in an article featured in the *Natural Medicine Review* (Fall 1998). "If you are like 55 percent of the population of the United States, you are overweight. And, if you are like 33 percent of the population, you are medically obese."

Statistics show that Americans are more than 60 percent deficient in vitamin B_6, magnesium, chromium, calcium, iron, zinc, and fiber. Other common deficiencies include vitamins A, C, B_1, B_2, B_{12}, and niacin. Most of these nutrients are considered essential because the body requires them in order to function properly. In addition, some estimates show that nearly 80 percent of the American population does not consume enough essential fatty acids (EFAs).

Carbohydrates   This category is made up of bone-building foods, as well as bone-damaging foods. Simple sugars are bone-damaging foods, while vegetables and whole grains are bone-building foods. Carbohydrates provide fuel for the body. Choose your carbohydrates wisely, and consume plenty of green, leafy vegetables. The more colorful the vegetable, the better it is for your bones and overall health. Sugar is detrimental to bone health because it increases calcium secretion. Studies have shown that as sugar intake increases, bone mass decreases.

Fats   The controversy surrounding fat intake has been building for years. By now we know there are "good" fats and "bad" fats. Fat is very important to the bones and overall health. Too much fat, on the other hand, can actually lower calcium levels in the body, contributing to osteoporosis. In addition, a high-fat diet has been linked to heart disease and cancer, the two biggest killer diseases in America. Saturated fats found in animal products and margarine, for example, are considered dangerous and should be reduced or avoided. In contrast, essential fatty acids (EFAs) and oils (such as flaxseed) have demonstrated a variety of health benefits. One study from the University of Pretoria, South Africa (*Prg Lipid Res*, Sept. 1997), reported that EFA-deficient animals developed severe osteoporosis. The researchers concluded: "EFAs have now been shown to increase calcium absorption from the gut, in part by enhancing the effects of vitamin D, to reduce urinary excretion of calcium, to increase calcium deposition in bone and improve bone strength, and to enhance the synthesis of bone collagen." The best advice about fat intake is to avoid margarine and use olive oil whenever possible, and try to get your fats from cold-water fish, such as cod, salmon, halibut, and tuna.

Protein We know that bones need protein to be strong; however, this is a prime example where more is not better. A diet with excess protein damages the bones. A high-protein diet can deplete calcium from the intestines. When calcium is excreted in this fashion, it is unavailable for bones. Without calcium, bones become porous and fragile. The type of protein is almost as important as the amount. Protein from animal sources seems to trigger a hormonal imbalance. A study featured in the *American Journal of Clinical Nutrition* (Sept 1988) followed vegetarian women and meat eaters for 20 years. At age 80, the meat eaters were found to have nearly twice the bone loss as their vegetarian counterparts. Of course, vegetarians get their protein from plant sources, such as nuts, seeds, beans, and tofu. We will discover later that certain plant foods also contain phytoestrogens, which may help balance hormones and fortify bone structure. In addition, green, leafy vegetables are rich in important natural antioxidants.

Specific dietary requirements

Now that we have some general guidelines on the three main dietary components, let's discuss specific dietary steps you can take to ensure optimum bone health. Remember, while diet is just one of the components of nature's bone-building plan, it is the foundation. It may not be necessary to follow the bone-building diet all the time, but the more you adhere to the plan, the better your chances of long-lasting bone health. Here are my top 10 bone-building dietary guidelines:

1. Eat plenty of green, leafy vegetables and colored foods, such as tomatoes and peppers. These foods are great sources of bone-building nutrients, such as calcium and vitamin K.

2. Eat other foods high in calcium, such as kale, cheddar cheese, seeds and nuts, yogurt (which all have more calcium than whole milk), olives, and broccoli. Magnesium—another vital bone-building mineral—is also found in these foods and others, including brown rice, avocados, and beans.

3. Reduce intake of animal fats and concentrate on the "good" fats found in fresh, cold-water fish; and olive, canola, evening primrose, and flaxseed oils.

4. Reduce sodium intake; it leaches calcium from bones.

5. Reduce or eliminate caffeine and carbonated drinks. Like salt, they sap vital calcium from the bones. Soft drinks are especially damaging to bone structure because they contain phosphates that interfere with calcium absorption. Drink more fresh water (at least eight 8-ounce glasses a day) and herbal teas.

6. Reduce or eliminate alcohol consumption. It, too, can disrupt calcium balance and cause excessive excretion of magnesium.

7. Reduce or eliminate sugar. This is another substance that drains the body of calcium.

8. Eat a moderate amount of protein and emphasize beans and fish as key sources. Balance is particularly important with protein, as both too little or too much can lead to poor bone health.

9. Eat organic foods whenever possible. There are no studies directly linking food additives and preservatives to osteoporosis, but we know these substances can interfere with optimum health.

10. Eat whole grains instead of refined flour. Refined grains lose a large percentage of their nutrient value during processing. It has been estimated that 60 percent of the calcium content and 85 percent of the magnesium content is lost in refined grains.

To help make appropriate food choices, refer to the table on the following page.

Good Sources Of...

Source	Serving	Amount

CALCIUM

Kelp	3.5 oz.	1,093 mg
Sesame seeds	.25 cup	500 mg
Turnip greens	1 cup	450 mg
Shrimp	1 cup	300 mg
Milk	1 cup	280 mg
Kale	3.5 oz.	250 mg
Almonds	3.5 oz.	234 mg
Soybeans	1 cup	130 mg
Pinto beans	1 cup	100 mg

MAGNESIUM

Cashews	3.5 oz	270 mg
Brown rice	3.5 oz	90 mg
Dried apricots	3.5 oz	60 mg
Prunes	3.5 oz	40 mg

VITAMIN K

Green tea	3.5 oz	700 mcg
Spinach	3.5 oz	400 mcg
Broccoli	3.5 oz	200 mcg
Asparagus	3.5 oz	60 mcg

VITAMIN D

Whole milk	1 quart	400 IU
Sun	30 min.	300 IU

Sources: USDA; *Encyclopedia of Nutritional Supplements* by Michael T. Murray, N.D.; *The Osteoporosis Solution* by Carl Germano, R.D.

Lifestyle factors

Research has confirmed that a wide variety of outside factors influence bone health. While diet is a big part of the picture, nature's bone-building program would not be complete without a thorough evaluation of your lifestyle. You can control lifestyle factors that influence the health of your bones. And again, these factors affect your bones long before the first fracture.

Let's begin by pinpointing the negative lifestyle factors, in addition to poor diet, that can drain bone strength and reduce bone mass.

<u>Smoking</u> We've already discussed how smoking can weaken bones and increase your risk of developing osteoporosis. This is definitely a direction worth repeating. If you smoke, you must find a way to quit. Absolutely no positive health benefits are associated with smoking. Let's add increased risk of developing osteoporosis to the long list of health dangers that can result from smoking.

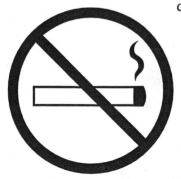

<u>Obesity</u> While it is true that women who carry a little extra body fat are at lower risk of developing osteoporosis, the extreme is not healthy either. Excess body fat can put undue pressure on bones and joints. Obesity has also been linked to heart disease and cancer. In addition, obesity can lead to a sedentary lifestyle, which is a key risk factor for developing osteoporosis.

Lack of knowledge Taking our bones for granted—not educating ourselves about the risks of developing osteoporosis and the ramifications of our lifestyles—is yet another negative factor that can lead to osteoporosis. It is vital to educate yourself and your family about the importance of bone health. As actress and women's health advocate Linda Evans has stated in her presentations on bone health, "We need to take responsibility for our health or we'll become a victim of our own lack of knowledge."

Exercise is a must

A wealth of scientific documentation demonstrates a direct link between physical activity and healthy bone structure. Here are some recent studies on exercise and bone health.

Animal study The effects of exercise on bone health at different ages were studied in Tokyo, Japan (*Tohoku J Exp Med*, May 1998). Five different groups of mice were put on different exercise programs at different ages. The researchers concluded that "exercise training at every age suppresses age-associated bone loss…"

Epidemiological study This type of study evaluates health patterns in a specific population. A Japanese study published in the *Journal of Epidemiology* (March 1998) evaluated more than 5,000 women from 14 different health centers throughout Japan. An evaluation of completed questionnaires showed a "beneficial influence of exercise on bone mineral density and its utility for preventing osteoporosis."

Meta-analysis When researchers review previously published studies, it's called a meta-analysis. *The Journal of American Geriatrics Society* (Feb 1998) featured a meta-analysis of ten studies evaluating the effects of aerobic exercise on spine bone density. The researcher concluded, "…aerobic exercise helps to maintain lumbar spine bone mineral density in postmenopausal women."

After reviewing much of the scientific literature, it is quite clear that the types of exercise providing the most benefit is weight bearing exercise. A Canadian study published in December 1997 (*Arch Phys Med Rehabil*) evaluated the effects of water exercise on bone mass. In the study, 77 women exercised in a pool with waist-high water for 60 minutes, three days a week, over a 12-month period. While functional fitness and psychological well-being improved, there was no effect on skeletal bone mass.

Walking seems to be one of the best forms of exercise to improve bone mass. And for more adventurous individuals, weight lifting can also provide benefit. A study featured in the *Journal of Sports Medicine and Physical Fitness* (Dec 1997) concluded that even a short-term weight training program can either maintain or improve bone mass density in premenopausal women.

In addition to walking and weight lifting, the National Osteoporosis Foundation recommends low-impact aerobics, skiing, hiking, tennis, and dancing. The goal is to be physically active. Even taking the stairs instead of the elevator, or parking farther away from the building entrance, can help. You may need to start out slow, but remember, every little bit helps!

Here are some general guidelines that will help you stick with your exercise program:

✔ If you have been inactive for a long time, it's a good idea to get a physical exam and some guidance from your doctor before beginning a new exercise program.
✔ Vary your activities to reduce the risk of boredom. And if you are going to try weight lifting, don't lift every day; your muscles need a chance to regenerate.
✔ Frequency is more important than intensity. Your program should provide some type of physical activity a minimum of three times per week.
✔ Duration and intensity are also important considerations. Try to exercise for a minimum of 30 minutes per session. Don't overdo it or you'll get frustrated and want to quit. The intensity of your workout should be based on your own limitations. Always stop if you are dizzy or experiencing pain.
✔ Moderation is also important, especially for younger women. Many studies have shown that some female athletes, especially those who are thin and fine-boned, who are involved in an intense exercise regimen, are at risk of losing bone mass. Typically, the first sign of a problem is if menstruation ceases or becomes irregular.

Yoga can also be an effective activity to incorporate into your routine. While yoga is not as physical as many activities, it promotes flexibility and helps the body relax. Wellness doctor Christiane Northrup, M.D., notices that her patients who practice yoga regularly seem to show the least height loss. Dr. Northrup states, "I believe that this is because yoga tends to keep the disc spaces between the vertebrae more supple and open."

No matter which exercise program or physical activity you participate in, be sure to wear comfortable, appropriate clothing, warm up and cool down, stretch before and after, and drink plenty of fresh water to keep muscles hydrated.

Exercise is perhaps the most powerful medicine available

to us today. It can help enhance self-image, alleviate depression and anxiety, and help prevent chronic, degenerative diseases like osteoporosis. It is a critical component of nature's bone-building plan.

If you're eating right and exercising, the final step toward optimum bone health for a lifetime involves specific nutrients found in nutritional supplements. But remember, just as the name implies, these products are "supplements." Nothing can replace a balanced diet, positive lifestyle habits, and consistent physical activity.

Bone-building nutrients

Just like your skin needs moisture to look healthy and vibrant, your bones need certain nutrients in order to remain strong. While a balance of essential vitamins and minerals is important, certain nutrients provide additional support for the bones. It is estimated that two dozen different nutrients have been identified as directly contributing to bone health. Minerals are most notably associated with bone health. Specifically, bone contains high concentrations of important minerals. It seems logical then that deficiencies in these minerals can result in bone problems.

Calcium The most well-known, clinically studied nutrient for bone health is the mineral calcium. This makes sense, considering that 99 percent of the total amount of calcium in our bodies is in our bones. It is the most abundant mineral in the human body. Bones require calcium to remain strong. The National Academy of Sciences recently increased the recommended calcium dosage to 1,000 mg of calcium per day for people ages 31 to 50, and 1,200 mg for ages 51 and older. The 1994 National Institutes of Health Optimal Calcium Intake Consensus recommends 1,500 mg for people over age 65. Calcium citrate is an easily absorbed form of calcium available in most over-the-counter supplements. Keep in mind that calcium must be balanced with magnesium. The ideal ratio of calcium to magnesium is 2:1. For example, if your nutritional supplement has 1,000 mg of calcium, it should contain 500 mg of magnesium.

Magnesium While calcium is important, some experts believe magnesium may be just as vital. According to holistic medical doctor and researcher Dr. Alan Gaby, magnesium deficiency appears to be one of the most widespread and clinically significant nutritional problems in the United States. We know that taking too much calcium can actually lead to a magnesium deficiency. About 60 percent of the magnesium in the human body is concentrated in the bones, while nearly 30 percent is in muscle tissue. Magnesium is important for energy production within the body, as it is involved in more than 300 enzymatic reactions. "Hardly a patient leaves my office without receiving a recommendation to take magnesium supplements," explains Dr. Gaby. Dr. Northrup warns, "A diet low in magnesium and relatively high in calcium can actually contribute to osteoporosis." It's another lesson in balance.

Zinc It has long been hypothesized that zinc deficiency can contribute to diminished bone tissue in athletes. A recent study at a medical hospital in Madrid, Spain (J Bone Miner Res, Mar 1998), confirmed these findings. Researchers concluded that zinc supplementation prevented the adverse effects of strenuous exercise on bone tissue in animals. Zinc's bone-building benefits could be explained by its intricate involvement in hormonal activity. In addition, high concentrations of zinc are present in bone tissue. Although the RDA for zinc is 12 mg for women and 15 mg for men, holistic healthcare practitioners often recommend as much as 30 mg.

<u>Boron</u>   Another key mineral for bone health is boron. Although we typically don't hear a lot about this trace mineral, it plays an important role in calcium and magnesium metabolism. Boron also works closely with vitamin D and hormones. There is no RDA for boron. Dr. Gaby recommends 0.5 to 3 mg of boron per day. Boron is found in high concentrations in fruits, vegetables, and nuts.

Two of the most important vitamins for bone health are vitamins D and K. Keep in mind, however, that **none of these nutrients are classified as approved treatments for osteoporosis.** They are dietary supplements that can help enhance bone health and bone tissue metabolism.

<u>Vitamin D</u>   When you're exposed to the sun, your body manufactures vitamin D. Besides the sun, we can get vitamin D from enriched milk, cold-water fish, and egg yolks. Vitamin D helps the body absorb calcium. The RDA for vitamin D for both men and women is 200 IU daily. However, higher amounts are often recommended for high-risk individuals (refer to risk assessment guide on page 80). Because vitamin D is fat soluble, it can potentially cause toxicity. Never exceed dosages of 1,000 IU per day, unless directed by your physician.

<u>Vitamin K</u>   This vitamin is intricately involved in bone health, as it helps produce a specific protein found in bone tissue. Without this protein, known as osteocalcin, bones would not have structure. They would be like chalk, fragile and easily broken. According to the 1995 *Annual Review of Nutrition,* "Several studies have demonstrated that a poor vitamin K status is associated with an increased risk of osteoporotic bone fractures." People who use antibiotics frequently face a higher risk of vitamin K deficiency. The medication destroys the friendly bacteria, which naturally produce vitamin K in the body. The RDA of vitamin K for an adult male is 80 mcg and for a female, 65 mcg. Holistic

medical doctors such as Dr. Gaby often recommend between 150 and 500 mcg per day. Vitamin K is found in green, leafy vegetables.

Science is discovering that vitamins and minerals are not the only substances that can benefit bone health.

It has long been known that plants contain powerful components with medicinal value. The study of herbal medicine has uncovered some potent, health-promoting substances. A good portion of today's prescription and over-the-counter drugs have their roots in herbal medicine.

Natural compounds found in plants, known as bioflavonoids and phytoestrogens, are receiving much attention from the scientific community. Some of these compounds are thought to provide therapeutic benefits for a wide range of conditions. The term phytoestrogen means that the plant has estrogenic activity.

I have a particular interest in a compound known as ipriflavone (pronounced i-pri-flay-vone). I have been so impressed with the research on this substance that I have devoted an entire chapter to it.

Test Your Knowledge...

TRUE OR FALSE?

Circle the appropriate response. Answers appear in the chapter highlights on the following page.

1. There is <u>no</u> connection between diet and bone health.

   True   False

2. Green, leafy vegetables are a great source of bone-building nutrients such as calcium and vitamin K.

   True   False

3. Cola drinks are especially bad for bone health.

   True   False

4. Water exercise is a good choice if you want to enhance bone strength.

   True   False

5. Never take calcium without taking magnesium.

   True   False

6. Nearly 100 percent of the body's calcium is concentrated in the bones.

   True   False

7. Boron is an approved drug for osteoporosis treatment in the United States.

   True   False

8. Exposure to sunlight creates vitamin D in the body.

   True   False

Chapter highlights:

- Measures can be taken to help maximize peak bone mass and minimize bone loss.
- The key to long-lasting bone health is to start as early as possible.
- Dietary factors play an important role in helping bones remain strong.
- Calcium is important, but it is not the only vital nutrient for bone health.
- A balanced diet, featuring plenty of fresh, colorful fruits and vegetables, is important.
- Sugar, sodium, caffeine, and alcohol can all deplete your bones of vital calcium.
- Do not smoke!
- Weight-bearing exercise is one of the most important factors for bone health.
- In addition to calcium, magnesium, zinc, boron, and vitamins D and K are important to bone health.
- These specific vitamins and minerals are not considered approved drugs for the treatment of osteoporosis.
- Substances in plants, called phytoestrogens/isoflavones, can contribute to bone health.

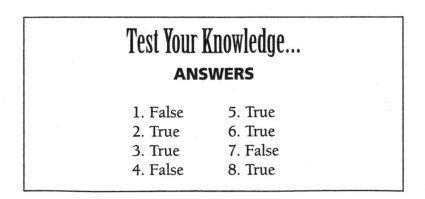

Test Your Knowledge...
ANSWERS

1. False	5. True
2. True	6. True
3. True	7. False
4. False	8. True

"...ipriflavone can...maximize bone mass while minimizing bone loss."

Chapter Four

IPRIFLAVONE—NATURE'S BONE BUILDER

It's been called the "alternative to estrogen" or the "new nutritional medicine" for osteoporosis. Ipriflavone is an isoflavone, which is a compound that naturally occurs in plants and foods. Isoflavones are ubiquitous in nature, meaning they are found virtually everywhere. Thanks to scientific advancements, we can now isolate and mass-produce ipriflavone.

Some researchers are calling ipriflavone the biggest breakthrough yet in osteoporosis prevention and treatment. I agree. It is the most thoroughly examined compound in the natural health field. Let's clarify one issue, however, before we begin discussing this exciting bone builder. Ipriflavone is not a cure. At this point, there is no known cure for osteoporosis.

On the other hand, preliminary studies report that ipriflavone can accomplish the two objectives of osteoporosis prevention and treatment: To maximize bone mass while minimizing bone loss.

In this chapter, we will learn that ipriflavone has been reported to:

✔ Stimulate calcitonin synthesis and secretion. Remember that calcitonin is the hormone, formed in the thyroid gland, that promotes calcium metabolism.
✔ Inhibit bone resorption (to slow down bone loss).
✔ Stimulate bone formation.
✔ Increase bone mineral density.
✔ Decrease fracture rate.
✔ Complement estrogen therapy.

A historical perspective

Ipriflavone is the abbreviated name for its proper chemical name, 7-isopropoxy isoflavone. The estrogenic effects of clover were discovered in cattle way back in the 1930s. In an effort to determine medicinal value, researchers began studying the variety of compounds within the plant kingdom, including isoflavones.

According to Steven Lee, research director with Technical Sourcing International, a Hungarian pharmaceutical company, actually isolated and discovered ipriflavone in 1969. Lee, who holds both MS and BS degrees in pharmacy, has studied ipriflavone extensively.

"In the early 1980s, pharmaceutical companies in Eastern Europe, Italy, and Japan started investigating ipriflavone's ability to enhance bone density," Lee explains. "Since the mid to late 1980s, ipriflavone has been an approved therapeutic agent for osteoporosis prevention and treatment in Europe and Japan."

Here's the ipriflavone time line:
1969 . . . . isolated and synthesized
1970 . . . . OTC product created
1974 . . . . animal studies
1981 . . . . human studies
1989 . . . . approved in 21 countries as a prescription for osteoporosis

Ipriflavone is found in larger quantities in alfalfa and propolis from bees. Although soy is a rich source of isoflavones, Steven Lee has clarified that the isoflavones in soy are primarily genistein and daidzein, not ipriflavone. According to Lee, a Japanese soy manufacturing company has attempted to isolate ipriflavone from soy but has been unsuccessful.

Today, ipriflavone is sold as an ingredient in dietary supplement formulas throughout the United States. Because it is not an approved drug, manufacturers are not allowed to make claims that the product treats osteoporosis.

I am often asked why ipriflavone is not an approved drug for the treatment of osteoporosis in the United States. Our drug approval process is much different than that of European countries. The cost of drug approval in the United States for a new chemical entity is now approaching $450 million and requires 12 to 15 years of development. Then, because ipriflavone is a natural substance that cannot be patented, and can easily be duplicated, any other manufacturer would be allowed to sell it as a drug without spending the time or money. Fortunately, European and US standards are getting closer, thanks to the efforts of the International Commission of Harmonization, whose goal it is to bring some consistency to the drug approval process throughout the world.

A scientific perspective

What impressed me most about ipriflavone is the strong scientific substantiation. My research on ipriflavone uncovered the following:

✔ More than 16 randomized, placebo-controlled human studies have been conducted, with one directly comparing ipriflavone to calcitonin.
✔ All of those studies demonstrated maintenance or an increase in bone mineral density.
✔ Two studies that examined fracture rate demonstrated a decrease in fracture rate.
✔ A total of 60 different clinical studies have been performed in Italy, Japan, and Hungary, involving nearly 2,800 patients with established osteoporosis.
✔ At the end of 1998, a large European multicenter trial for fracture prevention was being completed.

A search of the scientific literature reveals dozens of articles written about ipriflavone for bone health. I would like to briefly describe some of the more recent ones.

University of Siena, Italy (*Calcif Tissue Int*, Suppl 1997) This two-year study involved 111 elderly osteoporotic women, ages 65 to 79. Researchers concluded, "...long-term treatment with ipriflavone may be considered safe, and may increase bone density and possibly prevent fractures in elderly patients with established osteoporosis."

University of Siena, Italy (*Calcif Tissue Int*, Suppl 1997) This study involved 453 postmenopausal women (PMW), ages 50 to 65 years. Researchers concluded, "The compliance to the oral long-term treatment was good...ipriflavone is able to prevent both axial and peripheral bone loss in PMW with low bone mass, and is well tolerated."

Washington University School of Medicine, Missouri (*Calcif Tissue Int*, Suppl 1997) This animal study showed that after one month of treatment with ipriflavone, bone density was increased without altering mineral composition of bone tissue.

University of Pisa, Italy (*Maturitas*, Sep 1997) This two-year study focused on postmenopausal women. Study participants either received calcium alone, ipriflavone with calcium, low-dose conjugated estrogen, or ipriflavone with low-dose conjugated estrogen. Study results demonstrated that "Postmenopausal ipriflavone administration...can prevent the increase in bone turnover and the decrease in bone density that follows ovarian failure." The same was true for the combination therapy of ipriflavone and low-dose conjugated estrogen therapy.

Kyushu University, Japan (*Int J Gynaecol Obstet*, July 1998) This study specifically used conjugated equine (horse) estrogen therapy combined with ipriflavone in women during the first year following an oophorectomy (removal of the ovaries). The study found that use of ipriflavone with conjugated equine estrogen therapy, from an early stage after the surgery, inhibited bone loss and "was considered to be effective in maintaining bone mass after oophorectomy."

University of Siena, Italy (*Menopause*, Spring 1998) This study involved 56 women, less than five years into menopause, who had low vertebral bone density. Women taking just calcium had a decline in bone density after two years. However, bone density did not change in the women receiving ipriflavone and 1,000 mg of calcium daily. The researchers concluded, "Ipriflavone prevents the rapid bone loss following early menopause. This effect is associated with a reduction of bone turnover rate."

Equally as important as the published scientific studies, are the experiences physicians are witnessing in clinical practice. Many doctors throughout the world are seeing positive clinical results with their patients who are taking ipriflavone.

Dr. Susan Brown recommends using ipriflavone when diet and lifestyle factors don't provide the desired results. She prefers ipriflavone over the prescription drugs now available. She is currently conducting various ipriflavone pilot studies at the Osteoporosis Education Project in East Syracuse, New York. "Ipriflavone is being used as an adjunct therapy for those who require a stronger program to limit bone breakdown and enhance bone formation," she explains. "Ipriflavone holds more promise as a safe and effective bone-building agent than the drugs presently being used."

Ronald Hoffman, M.D., medical director of the Hoffman Center in New York City and host of his own popular radio program, also has many success stories with ipriflavone.

"I use ipriflavone as either an adjunct to medical treatments such as Fosamax or estrogen, or as a stand-alone treatment," explains Dr. Hoffman. "Ipriflavone works specifically on bone receptors and is very safe. I have used it on hundreds of patients."

Dr. Hoffman describes a recent success story involving a 55-year-old patient who had trouble with conventional medicine. The patient had a history of breast cancer, so she could not take estrogen. She also experienced side effects with the other medications available. "That left us with only ipriflavone and the other synergistic nutrients and lifestyle factors," Dr. Hoffman explained. Her initial bone density test confirmed that she had osteoporosis. After one year of treatment with ipriflavone, her bone density increased by nine percent.

"Ipriflavone is best when used with a balanced program that features other synergistic nutrients, such as calcium, magnesium, boron, silica, vitamin K, and others," concludes Dr. Hoffman.

The estrogen issue

Estrogen therapy is probably the most confusing, misunderstood issue in women's healthcare today. There are not enough pages in this book to thoroughly cover the topic of hormone replacement therapy (HRT). And besides, the purpose of this book is to help you evaluate your choices on bone health and the prevention of osteoporosis. Your decision whether to use HRT is one you should make after you have evaluated all of the information and applied it to your particular situation.

Is ipriflavone a good alternative to estrogen, specifically regarding bone health? Yes. For women who cannot tolerate the side effects of estrogen, or are concerned about the long-term risk of developing cancer, ipriflavone provides an effective alternative.

Keep in mind, however, that ipriflavone has only been studied on bone health. The effects of ipriflavone on menopausal symptoms such as hot flashes, night sweats, and others, is not known at this time. There have been no studies testing ipriflavone on menopausal symptoms. This is an area that may receive scientific exploration in the future.

Some studies have also shown that ipriflavone can act as an effective complementary therapy with HRT for the purpose of maintaining bone mass. If you are using ipriflavone this way, be aware that it will probably allow you to reduce your dosage of estrogen. However, never adjust your HRT dosage or discontinue your prescription without first consulting your doctor. HRT should be gradually reduced.

"We know that hormones like estrogen are very effective in the treatment of osteoporosis," explains Steve Lee. "A key disadvantage of hormone replacement therapy is that it may increase the risk of developing uterine and breast cancer."

"Ipriflavone, on the contrary, does not act on the hormone-bound receptors in the body at all," according to Lee. "The beauty of ipriflavone is that it inhibits bone resorption and stimulates bone formation."

Researchers at the University of Berne, Switzerland, showed in a clinical study that while ipriflavone "mimics the osteoprotective effect of estrogen...(its) lack of uterotropic (i.e., affecting the uterus) effect suggest that the compound can discriminate between bone and reproductive tissues."

The chemical structure of ipriflavone and estrogen are very similar. The difference is in how the body metabolizes each one. Hormone structure, function, and metabolism are complex topics. It is an area of medicine that will continue to be analyzed and researched for decades to come.

Hormones, and the natural substances that affect them, are powerful substances that should be treated with respect. More is not always better.

Is ipriflavone safe?

We all know that just because something is labeled "natural" doesn't necessarily mean it's safe. For example, tobacco is natural, and we know that's not safe. Obviously, while effectiveness is important, safety is just as critical.

Fortunately, ipriflavone seems to be both effective *and* safe. In all of the studies, oral ipriflavone was well tolerated. Some minor gastrointestinal discomfort was reported; however, it was equal to that of the placebo group (i.e., the subjects receiving a fake pill).

Because ipriflavone is metabolized in the liver, people with liver disease or weaknesses would not be good candidates for this supplement. We are also not sure how ipriflavone interacts with other medications that are metabolized in the liver, like oral contraceptives, epilepsy medications, some tranquilizers, and some antidepressants.

Certainly, when you compare ipriflavone to the drugs presently on the market for osteoporosis, it has fewer side effects.

The recommended dosage of ipriflavone is 600 mg daily in divided doses (200 mg three times daily). It is best absorbed when taken with food. When taken with a meal, 90 percent of ipriflavone is absorbed. There is no indication that more than 600 mg is ever required.

While side effects associated with long-term use of ipriflavone are not known, all indications are that this substance is safe for adults and even teenagers. At this point, it is not recommended for small children.

Ipriflavone is a popular bone-building ingredient in a variety of nutritional supplements designed to enhance bone health. Look for ipriflavone on the label of the product you purchase.

Test Your Knowledge...

TRUE OR FALSE?

Circle the appropriate response. Answers appear in the chapter highlights on the following page.

1. Ipriflavone is a component of isoflavones that are found in plants and foods.
   True   False

2. Ipriflavone is an approved treatment for osteoporosis in Europe.
   True   False

3. There have been no human clinical studies done using ipriflavone.
   True   False

4. Ipriflavone actually helps build bone tissue and inhibits the breakdown of bone tissue.
   True   False

5. Ipriflavone can be taken with estrogen.
   True   False

6. Ipriflavone has many side effects.
   True   False

7. Ipriflavone should be taken with meals.
   True   False

8. In the U.S., ipriflavone is a supplement, not a drug.
   True   False

Chapter highlights:

- While ipriflavone is not a cure for osteoporosis, it is one of the biggest breakthroughs in the area of osteoporosis prevention and treatment.
- Ipriflavone works on many different levels to help contribute to bone health.
- Ipriflavone is used as an approved pharmaceutical agent for the prevention and treatment of osteoporosis in many European countries.
- In the United States, ipriflavone is sold as an ingredient in dietary supplements available over-the-counter.
- A total of 60 different clinical studies have confirmed the safety and effectiveness of ipriflavone.
- Many physicians in the United States have reported positive clinical results with their patients who have osteoporosis or low bone density.
- Ipriflavone is a good alternative to estrogen for bone health in those women who cannot tolerate or do not want to take estrogen.
- Ipriflavone appears to be safe when taken at the recommended dosage, which is 600 mg daily in divided doses.

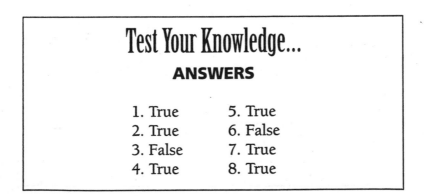

Test Your Knowledge...
ANSWERS

1. True	5. True
2. True	6. False
3. False	7. True
4. True	8. True

"...an effective bone-building program should include mind/body concepts."

Chapter Five

STOP OSTEOPOROSIS!

We've all seen the images: An individual slumped over, unable to even look up when her name is called; shuffling gingerly so as not to risk a fall; crippled and deformed. These are the agonizing results of osteoporosis. Pain, fear, and sadness accompany this disease into its advanced stages.

You may remember breaking a bone as a young child. You remember the discomfort and the inconvenience. You may even remember excruciating pain, or missing out on an important event because of your broken bone. However, we usually heal fast and bounce back quickly when we're young. But, imagine living with the fear of breaking a bone every day of your life. This is the life of a person with advanced osteoporosis. As the condition progresses, it's nearly impossible to live independently.

Osteoporosis is the extreme on the bone health continuum. On the opposite end of the spectrum is vitality, activity, and strength. This is the side of the continuum we want to be on—the end of the spectrum we strive for.

Osteoporosis is not an inevitable part of the aging process as previously thought. Even if you have a genetic predisposition, you can control many factors that lead to this devastating condition. Research has shown us that osteoporosis can be prevented.

And yet, at the rate this condition is growing, one-half of the adult female population will eventually succumb to osteoporosis. However, by following a comprehensive prevention plan that can also be used to complement osteoporosis treatment, you can beat the odds and defy the statisticians.

Get a head start

The sooner you begin your individual bone-building program, the better off you will be. Start early and teach your children about the importance of bone health.

"Osteoporosis is a largely preventable and treatable disease, and calcium is one critically important factor. But prevention should start in childhood and continue through our lives, not only with a high calcium intake and vitamin D, but also with weight-bearing exercise and a healthy lifestyle with no smoking and limited alcohol consumption," explains Felicia Cosman, M.D., clinical director of the National Osteoporosis Foundation.

And, it's not too late for those of you over the age of 50. You, too, can enhance your bone health with the concepts presented in this book. Remember, longevity experts predict that the average life expectancy of today's baby boomer will be nearly 100 years old. And our children are expected to live even longer. The question is, will we live to a ripe old age, leading an active, vibrant life, or will we be saddled with a chronic degenerative condition, such as osteoporosis? It's really never too late to enhance bone health, even if you've already been diagnosed with osteoporosis and are experiencing the traumatic symptoms of this condition.

Osteoporosis has been called the "silent disease." It could also be referred to as the "sideline disease," because victims of this condition are forced to sit on the sidelines of life, physically unable to fully participate.

A comprehensive prevention program should concentrate on getting rid of the silence. Discuss bone health with your doctor, your friends, and your children. Educate yourself and share the information with others.

The final key component to a comprehensive bone-building program involves a powerful medicine that doesn't come in a bottle. You can't find it at the grocery store or your local health club. This medicine is in each one of us and it's called attitude. Best of all, it's free!

Attitude is everything

There is an entire division of medicine known as psychoneuroimmunology. This is the study of how thoughts and feelings affect the immune system. Historically, medicine has kept mind and body separate, and has dismissed the health connection between the two. Today, we are recognizing the great power in the human brain that can help us enhance our physical health.

A growing body of scientific documentation connects thoughts and feelings to physical health. In October 1996, *The New England Journal of Medicine* reported that bone loss is greater in women who are depressed. The researchers studied 48 women with an average age of 41. They concluded, "The prominence of the deficits seen in these relatively young patients suggests that the lifetime risk of fracture related to depression is substantial."

It only makes sense that an effective bone-building program should include mind/body concepts. Here are some mind/body approaches to consider:

- ✔ **Positive attitude.** A positive attitude creates positive energy. Remember the last time you were with someone with a negative attitude? How did you feel after your visit? Probably drained. In contrast, when the "glass is half full," you find your outlook on life and your health often improve.
- ✔ **Spirituality.** For you, this may equate to a specific religion, a "higher power," or simply an enhanced spiritual connection to the world around you. Whatever you wish to call it, a strong spiritual influence in your life may have profound positive effects on your health.
- ✔ **Visualization.** Many people equate these techniques with cancer treatment. We hear stories of cancer patients who visualize Pac Man eating their cancer cells. Why can't this be true of many illnesses, including osteoporosis? Visualize a construction crew inside

your bones building new, healthy bone tissue. While I have no scientific evidence that this will actually help, I know that it will not hurt. You've got nothing to lose!

Other techniques used to help connect the mind with the body for better health include:

✔ Meditation and deep breathing exercises;
✔ Massage and body work (i.e., reiki, rolfing);
✔ Music therapy;
✔ Yoga and other "mindful" exercise programs;
✔ Laughter (remember, it's "the best medicine"); smile frequently and have fun;
✔ Love and support.

Surround yourself with loving people who support your health values and needs. Studies report that people who feel loved, and have a solid support system of family and friends, have a better chance of preserving or reclaiming good health.

According to a meta-analysis featured in the *American Journal of Psychiatry* (Jan 1997), researchers found that heart patients who were depressed, lonely, and felt isolated were 3.5 times more likely to die than their emotionally healthy counterparts. The idea of love and heart disease is quite an appropriate image.

Dr. Dean Ornish is one of the most well-known proponents of the mind/body connection. While his work has been done mostly with heart patients, he believes the concept can extend to other chronic diseases as well. "The real epidemic in our culture is depression, loneliness, and isolation," he says. "When our need for connection is unfulfilled, there are serious consequences not only in quality of life but in quantity of life."

Mind/body medicine sends a powerful message: Not only do your feelings and actions affect your health negatively or positively, so do the feelings and actions of those around you. Be careful with whom you associate.

Let's review...

The main message of this book is certainly worth repeating: The most successful bone-building/osteoporosis prevention program features a comprehensive attack. The battle plan should include:

❶ **Diet.** Omit items that can decrease bone mass, and incorporate more items that will enhance bone health.

❷ **Lifestyle factors.** Many activities that are well within your control can actually contribute to bone loss. The opposite is also true. Many activities, especially exercise, will positively contribute to bone health.

❸ **Nutrients.** While dozens of nutrients are specifically necessary for optimum bone health, special attention should be paid to calcium, magnesium, boron, and vitamins K and D.

❹ **Ipriflavone.** This substance shows great promise in the prevention and possible treatment of osteoporosis. Preliminary studies are very strong and the scientific community is giving this substance some well-deserved attention.

❺ **Attitude.** Science is confirming what many of us already know: When we support the mind and spirit, we support our physical health, too.

Ipriflavone questions and answers

To help clarify some important issues about ipriflavone, here are some common questions I am frequently asked:

Q. If I don't have osteoporosis or low bone mass, can I take ipriflavone as a preventive measure?

A. Absolutely. Ipriflavone, taken at the recommended dosage, is an ideal substance to help prevent osteoporosis, especially in high-risk individuals. Keep in mind, however, that there are no guarantees.

Q. If I already have osteoporosis, should I take more than the recommended daily amount?

A. No. All the studies thus far have used a dosage of 600 mg daily. There is no indication that more ipriflavone is better, or that the dosage depends on the stage of the condition. When dealing with dietary supplements, it's usually best to stick with the recommended dosage described on the label.

Q. Do I look for a product that contains just ipriflavone?

A. Ipriflavone is an ingredient included in many bone-building supplements. Look at the ingredient panel on the label to be sure the product contains ipriflavone in the form of 7-isopropoxy isoflavone. Many of the bone-building formulas on the market today have combined ipriflavone with other synergistic bone-building nutrients like calcium, vitamin K, and others. This makes sense. These bone-building supplements with ipriflavone are available over-the-counter, without a prescription. Ipriflavone is also sold alone, without added nutrients.

Q. Can I take ipriflavone if I am taking estrogen?

A. Yes. In fact, some studies have shown that ipriflavone actually enhances the effectiveness of estrogen. Be sure to tell your doctor that you are taking ipriflavone because you may be able to reduce your dosage of estrogen. Remember, however, that you should never stop taking estrogen or reduce your dosage without first consulting your doctor.

Q. Can I take ipriflavone if I am taking Fosamax?

A. Yes. However, patients typically choose one or the other. It is not necessary to take them both. If you can tolerate the Fosamax, you don't need the ipriflavone.

Q. What if my doctor does not feel I should be taking ipriflavone?

A. Your doctor may be hesitant because ipriflavone is a dietary supplement that has not been approved by the FDA as a drug for osteoporosis. I suggest you give your doctor this book. You may also want to provide him/her with other literature you can find on this subject. There is a complete listing of references at the back of this book. As more scientific information becomes available in the conventional medical literature about the clinical efficacy of ipriflavone, your doctor will become more aware of this substance. Until then, you may have to contribute some of the information. Don't be discouraged. Your doctor is just trying to protect your bone health as best he/she can, given the information available. And remember, your doctor will probably agree with the dietary and lifestyle recommendations in this book. Start by making those changes and your doctor will see how serious you are about this issue.

Q. A friend of mine started taking a product with ipriflavone and said she developed gastrointestinal problems. Is this common and should I be worried about this?

A. Some people experience some gastrointestinal upset with ipriflavone; however, usually taking the product with food will most likely eliminate this problem. If it persists, you may want to consider another product. Dr. Hoffman has said that he has treated hundreds of patients with ipriflavone and the compliance is quite high—meaning his patients stick with the supplement. Very few of his patients have experienced side effects with ipriflavone treatment.

Q. I eat a lot of soy to keep my hot flashes in check. Will ipriflavone help with that?

A. There are no studies showing that ipriflavone will provide any relief for menopausal symptoms such as hot flashes. While ipriflavone is an isoflavone, it has only been shown to specifically improve bone density. While there are many epidemiological studies demonstrating that soy can relieve hot flashes, to my knowledge, there are no studies underway to judge the effectiveness of ipriflavone on menopausal symptoms. Without that clinical data, we cannot confidently recommend ipriflavone for relief of menopausal symptoms such as hot flashes. At this point, researchers are pleased with the positive effects ipriflavone has on bone health. Perhaps in the future they will broaden their focus to include other conditions such as menopause. In the meantime, I suggest you continue eating soy foods.

Q. Should my 16-year-old daughter be taking ipriflavone?

A. Here are the circumstances under which I recommend ipriflavone for teenage girls:

1. If she is not eating a diet high in bone-building nutrients such as calcium, magnesium, and vitamins K and D.
2. If she is petite, small-boned, and exercises a lot (especially if she participates in intense athletics).
3. If you have a strong family history of osteoporosis. A strong family history is determined if a parent or grandparent has had the condition.

In each of these cases, it makes sense to supplement the diet with a bone-building formula that contains ipriflavone.

Final thoughts

It's shocking to consider how prevalent osteoporosis is. And it's not surprising that women especially are concerned about bone health.

"After menopause, a major part of a woman's adult life still lies ahead," states the National Osteoporosis Foundation. "To increase your chances of staying healthy, you have an important goal—to prevent bone loss."

There was a time when a woman was simply directed to get some exercise, take extra calcium, and see her doctor if a problem developed. Today, we've learned that a more proactive, comprehensive approach is necessary to prevent osteoporosis.

Osteoporosis is preventable. In addition to paying close attention to diet, lifestyle factors, and dietary supplements, it is important that you are aware of your individual risk factors. Complete the risk assessment questionnaire in Appendix II to get a clearer picture of your specific situation. In addition, ask your doctor about bone health during your next annual exam. Your doctor may recommend a bone density test. You will also want to pay close attention to your height as you age. Remember, if you lose more than two inches, you may be experiencing vertebral fractures. Talk to your doctor if you notice this bone loss.

If you already have osteoporosis, utilizing a comprehensive treatment plan will help you live an active, comfortable life. For best results, incorporate the concepts discussed in this book in your treatment program, if you are not already doing so.

Your bones deserve your attention. Just as you try to prevent heart disease, cancer, and the many other ills of our day, you should try to prevent osteoporosis. This condition can rob you of your independence and steal your vitality. Don't let yourself succumb to this silent epidemic. It's time to fight back!

Appendix I

RESOURCES

❶ The Osteoporosis Education Project
605 Franklin Park Dr.
East Syracuse, NY 13057
phone (315) 432-9231
fax (315) 463-7706
www.betterbones.com

The Osteoporosis Education Project is a research and education organization dedicated to the development of natural programs for the regeneration of bone health worldwide. The Project believes that every intervention or therapy dedicated to improving bone health should be good for the entire body: Better bones promote better bodies and better health. The Osteoporosis Education Project is privately funded through consulting and lecture services, supplemented by the sale of books and select products. The Osteoporosis Education Project is directed by Dr. Susan E. Brown, medical anthropologist and certified clinical nutritionist.

SPECIAL NOTE: To support the efforts of this important program, a portion of the proceeds from the sale of this book will be donated to The Osteoporosis Education Project.

❷ National Osteoporosis Foundation
1150 17th St., N.W., Suite 500
Washington, DC 20036-4603
phone (202) 223-2226
fax (202) 223-2237
www.nof.org

The National Osteoporosis Foundation is the nation's leading source of up-to-date, medically sound educational materials for patients and healthcare professionals on the causes, prevention, detection, and treatment of osteoporosis. It is the only scientific and medically based nonprofit, voluntary health organization devoted to osteoporosis.

Appendix II

RISK ASSESSMENT GUIDE

Prevention is the most critical component of the bone-building program outlined in this book. To help you reduce your risk of developing osteoporosis, I have developed this easy-to-use risk assessment questionnaire. Simply circle "yes" or "no," based on your individual situation. The more "yes" answers you have, the greater your risk is of developing this serious condition. You should discuss your answers with your doctor to determine an effective bone density evaluation program, and outline an individualized osteoporosis prevention or treatment plan.

● Are you small-boned and petite?　　yes　　no

● Are you Caucasian or Asian?　　　yes　　no

● Do you *seldom** walk, jog, or
　are involved in physical activity?　yes　　no
　(*less than 1 to 2 times per week)

● Are you menopausal?　　　　　　yes　　no

● Have you had surgically-induced
　menopause?　　　　　　　　　　yes　　no

● Do you smoke?   yes   no

● Does a member of your immediate
   family have osteoporosis?   yes   no

● Have you used a corticosteroid
   (i.e., Prednisone) for a long period? yes   no

● Do you drink more than three
   glasses of alcohol per week?   yes   no

● Do you drink more than one cup
   of coffee per day?   yes   no

● Do you *seldom* get sunshine?   yes   no

● Do you drink soft drinks regularly? yes   no

● Do you eat red meat every day?   yes   no

● Do you eat *few* green vegetables?   yes   no

● Have you experienced long
   bouts of depression?   yes   no

Total number of "yes" answers: _____

References

1. Acerbi D, Poli G, Ventura P: Comparative bioavailability of two oral formulations of ipriflavone in health volunteers at steady-state. Eur J Drug Metab Pharmacokinet 23(2):172-7, Apr/Jun 1998.
2. Agnusdei D, Bufalino L: Efficacy of ipriflavone in established osteoporosis and long-term safety. Calcif Tissue Int Suppl 61 1:23-27, 1997.
3. Agnusdei D, Crepaldi G, Isaia G, Mazzuoli G, Ortolani S, Passeri M, Bufalino L, Gennari C: A double-blind, placebo-controlled trial of ipriflavone for prevention of postmenopausal spinal bone loss. Calcif Tissue Int 61(2):142-147, Aug 1997.
4. Ahlgrimm M, Kells J: Restoring Balance: An Individualized Approach to Hormone Replacement Therapy. Green Bay: IMPAKT Communications, Inc., 1998.
5. Alternative Medicine: The Definitive Guide. Puyallup: Future Medicine Publishing, 1994.
6. Ames M: Are you overfed and undernourished? Natural Medicine Review, Fall 1998.
7. Anagnostakos NP, Tortora GJ: Principles of Anatomy and Physiology, Fifth Edition. New York: Harper & Row, 1987.
8. Anonymous: Caffeine associated with higher risk of hip fracture. Geriatrics 46(3):18, 1991.
9. Arky R (medical consultant): Physician's Desk Reference, 52nd Edition. Montvale: Medical Economics Company, 1998.
10. Brandi ML: Natural and synthetic isoflavones in the prevention and treatment of chronic diseases. Calcif Tissue Int Suppl 61, 1:5-8, 1997.

11. Bravo G, Gauthier P, Roy PM, Payette H, Gaulin P: A weight-bearing, water-based exercise program for osteopenic women: Its impact on bone, functional fitness, and well-being. *Arch Phys Med Rehabil* 78(12):1275-1380, Dec 1997.

12. Brown S, personal interview, March 1999, director, Osteoporosis Education Project, East Syracuse, NY.

13. Cheng SL, *et al*: Stimulation of human osteoblast differentiation and function by ipriflavone and its metabolites. *Calcif Tissue Int* 55(5):356-362, Nov 1994.

14. Choi YK, *et al*: Ipriflavone for the treatment of osteoporosis. *Osteoporosis Int* (Suppl 7) 1997.

15. Civitelli R: *In vitro* and *in vivo* effects of ipriflavone on bone formation and bone biomechanics. *Calcif Tissue Int* Suppl 61, 1:12-14 1997.

16. Cecchini MG, Fleisch H, Muhibauer RC: Ipriflavone inhibits bone resorption in intact and ovariectomized rats. *Calcif Tissue Int* Suppl 61, 1:9-11 1997.

17. Researchers say Fosamax may cause gastrointestinal problems. *Doctor's Guide to Medical and Other News*, Oct 1998.

18. deAloysio D, *et al*: Bone density changes in postmenopausal women with the administration of ipriflavone alone or in association with low-dose ERT. *Gynecol Endocrinol* 11(4):289-293, Aug 1997.

19. Dornemann TM, McMurray RG, Renner JB, Anderson JJ: Effects of high-intensity resistance exercise on bone mineral density and muscle strength of 40 to 50-year-old women. *J Sports Med Phys Fitness* 37(4):246-251, Dec 1997.

20. Edwards L, Fraser M: How do we increase awareness of osteoporosis? *Baillieres Clin Rheumatol* 11(3):631-644, Aug 1997.

21. Gaby AR: *Preventing and Reversing Osteoporosis*. Rocklin: Prima Publishing, 1994.

22. Gaby AR, Wright J: *Nutritional Therapy in Medical Practice*, Professional Seminar, Seattle, WA, Oct 1998.

23. Gambacciani M, Cappagli B, Piaggesi L, Ciaponi M, Genazzani AR: Ipriflavone prevents the loss of bone mass in pharmacological menopause induced by GnRH-agonists. *Calcif Tissue Int* Suppl 61 1:15-18, 1997.

24. Gambacciani M, Ciaponi M, Cappagli B, Piaggesi L, Genazzani AR: Effects of combined low dose of the isoflavone derivative ipriflavone and estrogen replacement on bone mineral density and metabolism in postmenopausal women. *Maturitas* 28(1):75-81, Sep 1997.

25. Gazella KA: Menopause: natural alternatives to conventional estrogen. *Nature's Impact*, Oct/Nov 1997.

26. Gennari C, Adami S, Agnusdei D, Bufalino L, Cervetti R, Crepaldi, DiMarco C, DiMunno O, Fantasia L, Isaia GC, Mazzuoli GF, Ortolani S, Passeri M, Serni U, Vecchiet L: Effect of chronic treatment with ipriflavone in postmenopausal women with low bone mass. *Calif Tissue Int* Suppl 61, 1:19-22, 1997.

27. Gennari C, Agnusdei D, Crepaldi G, Isaia G, Mazzuoli G, Ortolani S, Bufalino L, Passeri M: Effect of ipriflavone—a synthetic derivative of natural isoflavones—on bone mass loss in the early years after menopause. *Menopause* 5(1):9-15, Spring 1998.

28. Germano C: *The Osteoporosis Solution*. New York: Kensington, 1998.

29. Gossi M, *et al*: Inhibition of parathyroid hormone-stimulated resorption in cultured fetal rat long bones by the main metabolites of ipriflavone. *Calcif Tissue Int* 58(6):419-422, June 1996.

30. Glaser DL, Kaplan FS: Osteoporosis: definition and clinical presentation. *Spine* Suppl 24 22:12-16, Dec 1997.

31. Glassman AH, Shapiro PA: Depression and the course of coronary artery disease. *Am J Psychiatry* 155(1):4-11, Jan 1998.

32. Head KA: Ipriflavone: an important bone-building isoflavone. *Altern Med Rev* 4(1):10-22, Feb 1999.

33. Heersche JN, Bellows CG, Ishida Y: The decrease in bone mass associated with aging and menopause. *J Prosthet Dent* 79(1):14-16, Jan 1998.

34. Hoffman R, personal interview, Hoffman Center, New York, NY, March 1999.

35. Hoshi A, Watanabe H, Chiba M, Inaba Y: Effects of exercise at different ages on bone density and mechanical properties of femoral bone of aged mice. *Tohoku J Exp Med* 185(1):15-24, May 1998.

36. Hurley DL: Update on primary osteoporosis. *Mayo Clin Proc* 72(10):943-949, Oct 1997.
37. Kamen B: *Hormone Replacement Therapy: Yes or No?* Novato: Nutrition Encounter, 1998.
38. Kano K: Relationship between exercise and bone mineral density among over 5,000 women aged 40 years and above. *J Epidemiol* 8(1):28-32, Mar 1998.
39. Kelley G: Aerobic exercise and lumbar spine bone mineral density in postmenopausal women: a meta-analysis. *J Am Geriatr Soc* 46(2):143-152, Feb 1998.
40. Kleerekoper M: Detecting osteoporosis: beyond the history and physical examination. *Postgrad Med* 103(4):45-47, 51-52, 62-63, Apr 1998.
41. Kotkowiak L: Behavior of selected bio-elements in women with osteoporosis. *Ann Acad Med Stein* 43:225-238, 1997.
42. Kruger MC, Horrobin DF: Calcium metabolism, osteoporosis, and essential fatty acids: a review. *Prog Lipid Res* 36(2-3):131-151, Sep 1997.
43. Lee S, personal interview, March 1999.
44. Lehigh Valley Hospital and Health Network website.
45. Marsh AG, Sanchez TV, Michelsen O, Chaffee FL, Fagal SM: Vegetarian lifestyle and bone mineral density. *Am J Clin Nutr* (Suppl 3)48:837-841, Sept 1988.
46. Martini M, *et al*: Effects of ipriflavone on perialveolar bone formation. *Calcif Tissue Int* 63(4):312-319, Oct 1998.
47. *Merck Manual of Medical Information.* Whitehouse Station: Merck & Co., 1997.
48. Michelson D, Stratakis C, Hill L, Reynolds J, Galliven E, Chrousos G, Gold P: Bone mineral density in women with depression. *N Engl J Med* 335(16):1176-1181, Oct 1996.
49. Miller P, Lukert B, Broy S, Civitelli R, Fleischmann R, Gagel R, Khosla S, Lucas M, Maricic M, Pacifici R, Recker R, Sarran HS, Short B, Short MJ: Management of postmenopausal osteoporosis for primary care. *Menopause* 5(2):123-131, Summer 1998.
50. Miyauchi A, *et al*: Novel ipriflavone receptors coupled to calcium influx regulate osteoclast differentiation and function. *Endocrinology* 137(8):3544-3550, Aug 1996.

51. Murray MT: *Encyclopedia of Nutritional Supplements.* Rocklin: Prima Publishing, 1996.
52. National Institutes of Health Consensus Development Conference Statement, April 1984 (originally published in *Osteoporosis* 5(3):1-6).
53. National Osteoporosis Foundation website, www.nof.org.
54. Need AG, Morris HA, Horowitz M, Scopacasa E, Nordin BE: Intestinal calcium absorption in men with spinal osteoporosis. *Clin Endocrinol* (Oxf) 48(2):163-168, Feb 1998.
55. Northrup C: *Women's Bodies, Women's Wisdom.* New York: Bantam, 1995.
56. Notoya K, *et al*: Increase in femoral bone mass by ipriflavone alone and in combination with 1 alpha-hydroxy vitamin D3 in growing rats with skeletal unloading. *Calcif Tissue Int* 58(2):88-94, Feb 1996.
57. Nozaki M, Hashimoto K, Inoue Y, Ogata R, Okuma A, Nakano H: Treatment of bone loss in oophorectomized women with a combination of ipriflavone and conjugated equine estrogen. *Int J Gynaecol Obstet* 62(1):69-75, Jul 1998.
58. Osteoporosis and Related Bone Disease National Resource Center: *Smoking and Bone Health.* January 1998.
59. Reginster JY, Taquet AN, Gosset C: Therapy for osteoporosis: miscellaneous and experimental agents. *Endocrinol Metab Clin North Am* 27(2):453-63, June 1998.
60. Schachter M: The prevention of post-menopausal osteoporosis. *HealthWorld Online* (www.healthy.net).
61. Seco C, Revilla M, Herandez ER, Gervas J, Gonzalez-Riola J, Villa LF, Rico H: Effects of zinc supplementation on vertebral and femoral bone mass in rats on strenuous treadmill training exercise. *J Bone Miner Res* 13(3):508-512, Mar 1998.
62. *Taber's Cyclopedia Medical Dictionary.* Philadelphia: F.A. Davis, 1993.
63. Ushiroyama T, *et al*: Efficacy of ipriflavone and 1 alpha vitamin D therapy for the cessation of vertebral bone loss. *Int J Gynaecol Obstet* 48(3):283-288, Mar 1995.
64. Vassilopoulou-Sellin R, Brosnan P, Delpassand A, *et al*: Osteopenia in young adult survivors of childhood cancer. *Medical and Pediatric Oncology* 32:272-278, 1999.

65. Yamamoto Y, Kurabayashi T, Tojo Y, Yahata T, Honda A, Tomita M, Tanaka K: Effects of progestins on the metabolism of cancellous bone in aged oophorectomized rats. *Bone* 22(5):533-537, May 1998.

66. Wright JV, Morgenthaler J: *Natural Hormone Replacement.* Petaluma: Smart Publications, 1997.

Index

A

B

C

D

E

F

G

H

I

L

liver, 62
love, 70

M

magnesium
    general, 41, 48
    sources, 42
massage, 70
meditation, 70
menopause, 5, 9, 24, 60
Miacalcin (see parathyroid hormone)
mind/body, 68-70

N

National Institutes of Health, 1, 17, 47
National Osteoporosis Foundation, 2, 10, 21, 78
NTx Osteomark, 25

O

obesity, 43
oophorectomy, 58
organic, 41
osteoblast, 5, 7, 9
osteocalcin 49
osteoclast, 5, 7, 9, 12
osteopenia, 5, 25
osteoporosis
    conventional treatment for, 25, 27-30
    definition, 5, 17
    diagnosis, 25, 26
    diet, 37-42
    general, 17, 19, 21, 67
    lifestyle factors, 22, 23, 25, 43

T

testosterone, 12
thyroid, 22
tranquilizers, 62

U

ulcers, 28
urine test (see NTx Osteomark)

V

vegetarian, 40
vertebral fracture, 18
visualization, 69
vitamin D
        dosage, 49
        general, 39, 49
        sources, 42
vitamin K
        dosage, 49
        general, 40, 49
        sources, 42, 50

W

walking, 45
wrist fracture, 18

Y

yoga, 46, 70

Z

zinc, 48

Other booklets and books published by
IMPAKT Communications:

Booklets

• *Attention Deficit Disorder* by Jesse Lynn Hanley, M.D.
• *Build Strong Bones* by Angela Stengler, N.D., and
  Mark Stengler, N.D.
• *CoQ10* by Ray Sahelian, M.D.
• *Drink Your Greens* by Mark Stengler, N.D.
• *Heart Disease* by Karolyn A. Gazella, featuring an interview
  with Kilmer McCully, M.D.
• *Kava* by Ray Sahelian, M.D.
• *Lipoic Acid* by Ray Sahelian, M.D.
• *Menopause* by Angela Stengler, N.D., and Mark Stengler, N.D.
• *Osteoarthritis* by Karolyn A. Gazella, featuring an interview
  with Jason Theodasakis, M.D.
• *St. John's Wort* by Ray Sahelian, M.D.
• *Vanish Varicose Veins* by Sherry Torkos, B.Sc., Phm.
• *Your Child's Health* by Angela Stengler, N.D., and
  Mark Stengler, N.D.

Books

• *Activate Your Immune System* by Leonid Ber, M.D., and
  Karolyn A. Gazella
• *Buyer Be Wise! The Consumer's Guide to Buying Quality
  Nutritional Supplements* by Karolyn A. Gazella
• *Devour Disease with Shark Liver Oil* by Peter T. Pugliese, M.D.,
  with John Heinerman, Ph.D.

These booklets and books are available at your local health food
store or by calling 1-800-477-2995 (credit card orders only).

For a **free** list of

books and booklets

published by IMPAKT Communications, Inc.,

send the completed form to the address

below, or fax it to 1-920-434-8884.

IMPAKT Communications, Inc.
P.O. Box 12496
Green Bay, WI 54307-2496

Please send me a FREE list of your books and booklets!

FIRST NAME _____

LAST NAME _____

COMPANY (IF APPLICABLE) _____

MAILING ADDRESS _____

CITY _____ STATE _____ ZIP _____

PHONE ( ) _____ FAX ( ) _____

BBH99

I M PAKT
IMPAKT Communications

www.impakt.com